MANAGING THE CLINICAL RESOURCE

AN ACTION-GUIDE FOR HEALTH CARE PROFESSIONALS

ANNE JONES
and **UNA McDONNELL**

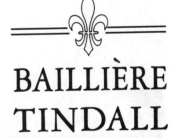

BAILLIÈRE TINDALL

LONDON PHILADELPHIA TORONTO SYDNEY TOKYO

Baillière Tindall
W.B. Saunders

24–28 Oval Road
London NW1 7DX

The Curtis Center
Independence Square West
Philadelphia, PA 19106 – 3399, USA

55 Horner Avenue
Toronto, Ontario, M8Z 4X6, Canada

Harcourt Brace & Company
(Australia) Pty Ltd
30–52 Smidmore Street
Marrickville
NSW 2204, Australia

Harcourt Brace Japan Inc
Ichibancho Central Building,
22–1 Ichibancho
Chiyoda-ku, Tokyo 102, Japan

© 1993 Baillière Tindall

This book is printed on acid-free paper

A catalogue record for this book is available from the British Library

ISBN 0–7020–1681–0

Typeset by Fakenham Photosetting Ltd, Fakenham, Norfolk
Printed and bound in Great Britain by Mackays of Chatham PLC, Chatham, Kent

MANAGING THE
CLINICAL RESOURCE

CONTENTS

CONTENTS

PREFACE

There is a wide selection of texts on management studies in which writers seek to act as exponents of management theory. Based on academic research new theories are developed and older ones adapted, compared and contrasted, in the light of new thinking and debate. The writers in this case are not attempting to produce an academic reference book. This text is not based on academic research or indeed an intensive search of available literature: rather, we seek to expose empirical evidence in order to give what is written a practical bias. It would be futile, however, to make any effort to produce such a project without reference to well tried and tested theories. However the maxim on which we based our early thoughts was that theory without practice is indeed futile, whilst practice without theory is blind. We hope at least to have achieved a balance.

This book is intended to illustrate management issues in professional practice in the light of contemporary thinking in the NHS as it celebrates 45 years as part of British social history. Clinicians and managers are challenged with the task of ensuring that the service is further developed to meet the needs of the British people as its consumers over the next decade and beyond. We have been party to many of the exciting challenges with which provider and purchaser agencies are currently involved. This book represents our keen interest in sharing some of the observations made during the course of gaining this rich experience.

Clinical services function as part of a broader external environment. The environment affects the service through, for example, technological and scientific development, economic activity, social and cultural influences, and governmental actions. The effect of the impact of these environmental influences on professionals is reflected in terms of the management of opportunities and risks, and successful achievement of its aims and objectives. The increasing rate of change in environmental factors has highlighted the need to manage the development of professional practice against a backcloth of dynamic change currently taking place within the NHS. Our main concern is not with the complex detail of the individual topic areas that form the basis of each chapter. What the book seeks to do is to provide an opportunity for readers to contextualize their own practice within the wider environment.

The use of separate topic areas is a recognized means of aiding study and explanation of the subject. However, in practice, the activities of professional practice and the job of managing professional resources cannot be neatly isolated into discrete categories. The majority of actions are likely to involve a number of simultaneous functions that relate to the total process of service delivery. The chapters in the book should not be regarded therefore as entirely freestanding. The underlying theme is the need for organizational effectiveness and the role professional practitioners have in effective organizations. Every work organization is concerned with being effective, especially now in a difficult economic climate. Effectiveness should be the concern of everyone within the organization. Only on attaining its aims and objectives will the organization be successful and ultimately remain viable.

The Government White Paper *Working for Patients*, published in January 1989, set out radical reforms for the NHS. A detailed discussion is inappropriate here, but a consideration of the essential philosophies is relevant. There is no greater test of the robustness of Resource Management than the introduction of *Working for Patients*. The White Paper proposed that Health Authorities, now known as Commissioning Authorities or Purchasers will effectively be searching for the best buy for their patients. The care may be obtained from existing NHS hospitals, Trust hospitals or community units or from the private sector. Purchasers and Providers will be cross-charged for their cross-boundary referral practices. A competitive market will be created and encouraged by the Government. Another aspect of the White Paper is the fundholding status of some General Practitioners (GPs). *Working for Patients* recognized that GPs were uniquely placed to improve patients' choice of good quality services because of their relationship with patients, hospitals and other members of the Primary Health Care Team. The principal aim of the GP Fundholding scheme is to build on this unique situation so that patients benefit further. It calls for the development of a management infrastructure and information handling capacity which enables large general practices to take control of expenditure on certain services delivered to their patients.

Chapter 1 provides an introduction to the concept of resource management. The Resource Management Initiative, a national project funded by the Department of Health, was initially implemented as an experiment in 1986 in six acute hospital sites in the UK. The initiative represents a complex project with a single aim – to allow total and individual patient care to be planned, delivered and costed effectively. This concept now forms a crucial part of the Government's plans for the future of the NHS both in hospital and community care.

An insight into the issue of health care economics is given in Chapter 2. The chapter is concerned with the application of economic analysis to management decisions. In the management of health care, there are decisions taken by non-economists, that is, managers, where the economist's approach can make a useful contribution. Central to this approach is an assessment of the costs and benefits associated with the alternative uses of resources. Economic principle applied to health care is the subject of emotive debate. The moral issue of fixing prices to health care might prove difficult for health care professionals to accept and internalize. However, all business decisions are concerned with the acquisition of resources, and where health care is concerned, the transformation of those resources into services to be supplied to customers of various types. The chapter is devoted to raising awareness of health care economics in the context of clinical service delivery.

Chapter 3 is given to the management of information and information technology. The NHS is undergoing dynamic change in the way that information is generated and subsequently used. Technology is being developed as a tool with which to process information so that managers can plan services and account for resource allocation. Credible and timely information is necessary to support decision-making which ultimately underpins service provision to patients and clients.

Chapter 4 is concerned with managing the human resource. Given that health care professionals represent the largest proportion of manpower in the service, the specific issues of skill mix and reprofiling are addressed here.

Chapter 5 addresses the management of change. Change is discussed in the context of organization development and the attempts at organic rather than cosmetic change. Change is perhaps the only aspect of organizations that remains constant. Notwithstanding, the criticism of clinicians is currently directed against the speed of the introduction of change rather than the actual amount. Inevitably, empirical evidence does not provide a prescription for change made easy, only a framework within which managers may work with creativity and flexibility.

Chapter 6 addresses the subject of project management as a methodology on which to base managerial practice. The writers' personal work experience within the project environment was the motivating factor for its inclusion. It may be a new concept for many clinicians but as an approach to management in everyday work situations it is a useful tool.

Chapter 7 provides a focus for quality. There is a strong emphasis in the NHS on quality care and very practical advice and help is becoming available in assessing and monitoring the quality of health care in it. However, the challenge faces all those involved in health care provision. The Citizen's Charter 'Raising the Standard' contains the assertion that 'better quality services do not happen by accident. Improvement requires reform, innovation and tough decisions'. There will be a continuation of central government lead, building on the developments in the NHS by the publication of charters in England, Scotland and Wales. These will spell out what the NHS should provide to meet people's needs at local level.

Finally Chapter 8 introduces the reader to marketing concepts. Commercial organizations have had well-developed marketing techniques with profit-making as a goal. The NHS as a public sector organization is not primarily profit-making. However the introduction of the reforms has created an internal market and the application of marketing concepts is now more appropriate than ever.

The book is designed to be of practical use to clinicians as much as to those in management and those aspiring to managerial positions. The target readership crosses the boundaries of professional disciplines. It should be noted that the terms clinician and health care professional are used interchangeably, both being ways of describing those practitioners who manage and provide patient/client contact. It is hoped that the work is user friendly and that clinicians can access the information in any order they find appropriate rather than reading from start to finish.

The chapters in the book are written to a standard format, whereby a brief introduction is followed by the identified aims for that chapter. This approach has been adopted in order to give an early indication of the topic areas covered, and also to enable readers to focus on their own specific learning outcomes as appropriate.

The Action Guidelines which are featured at the end of Chapters 2 to 8 highlight the salient points raised in the particular subject area. Questions are posed within these guidelines. The intention of this is to facilitate the transfer of the theoretical component into the context of actual clinical practice. We hope that these two features enhance the user friendliness of the book.

The issues discussed in the book are all part of an NHS agenda. They are part of a fundamental change in the service, the theme being that by improving the use and application of information, the gap that existed since 1948 will be bridged between the effective management of resources and the care of patients and clients.

ACKNOWLEDGEMENTS

It is customary for an author to extend thanks to all the people who helped with the book. The authors would like to begin by thanking the academic staff of the Health Service Management Unit at Manchester University and the Business School at the John Moores University of Liverpool respectively. During the course of study in these academic institutions the framework was provided within which much of the work for this publication was developed.

Our thanks are extended to all our colleagues in the hospital and community units throughout the Mersey Regional Health Authority. Our involvement with them and the learning experience gained from the Resource Management Programme has been invaluable and a rich influence on our writing. Thanks go to Pat Benning and John Prescott of the Aintree Hospitals NHS Trust in Liverpool for their specific contribution to the chapter on project management. Particular thanks are given to Les Gordon for his dedicated patience and technical advice in the preparation and final production of the manuscript.

Finally we would like to thank our families who gave us continued support and encouragement, and most of all, never doubted we would achieve the goal.

ANNE JONES
UNA MCDONNELL

PUBLISHER'S ACKNOWLEDGEMENTS

We would like to acknowledge the following organizations for permission to reproduce material from their publications.

Resource Management - Changing the Culture, one of a series of publications on organizational development by the NHS Training Directorate.

Total Quality Management, Carfax Publishing Company, Abingdon, Oxford.

Quality Improvement: The Role and Application of Research Methods, P. Batalden et al, Journal of Health Administration Education, Princeton University Press, N.J.

Confidential Enquiry into Maternal Deaths in England and Wales 1979-1981
The Citizens Charter, Raising the Standards, 1991
NHS Management Enquiry: The Griffiths Report 1983
Crown copyright, reproduced with the permission of Her Majesty's Stationery Office.

Special thanks to the Institute of Health Service Managers for permission to reproduce material from their publications *Change and Innovation*, and *Health Services Management*, April 1989.

RESOURCE MANAGEMENT

1

As we progress through a new era of health care management, perhaps the most significant change is one of focus. In the past, health care management was geared to the purpose of maintaining the organization. With the implementation of major change in the NHS, resource management, the Patient's Charter and continuous quality improvement programmes, the 'process' of patient care has become central to current information and management arrangements. Clinicians (doctors, nurses and the professions allied to medicine) have become actively involved in management to ensure that decisions are taken with the patient as the primary focus.

CHAPTER AIMS

☐ To set the topic of resource use into the context of the current NHS management climate

---

CONTEXT

Clinicians have always had a role in management, albeit perhaps a less explicit one than will be the case in future. It is now essential to develop health care professionals as corporate operators to enable them to work within the context of the organization and multidisciplinary group, rather than to work solely within their own discipline. This is particularly important to ensure that they continue to enhance their professional role, but also to enable them to influence activities and developments throughout the whole organization. A key task for the professions will be the positioning of effective clinical leaders in management which will ensure that present and future organization plans are more responsive to the needs of patients.

The NHS is a service organization, and there is now a greater emphasis placed on understanding the nature of the service's operations, and its outputs and outcomes in relation to the mix of resources used to provide those services. Service delivery and consumption occur simultaneously and so the needs and demands of those using the service must be central to its management and future development.

The Resource Management Initiative in the National Health Service

The Resource Management Initiative, a national project funded by the Department of Health, was initiated in 1986 at six experimental sites in England. The initiative represents a complex project with a single aim – to allow total patient care and its quality to be planned, delivered and costed effectively. This concept now forms a crucial part of the Government's plans for the future of the NHS.

The health service has traditionally planned and controlled its activities on a functional basis – monitoring what is spent on nursing, physiotherapy, or pathology, for example. Specialty costing has been introduced allowing costs of particular services to be established along with an average cost for treatment of patients. An average patient cost, however, can make no allowance for the complexity of treatment, the severity of the patient's condition, age or general state of health. The sensible planning of patient care thus becomes very difficult. Resource management is intended to address these deficiencies. In the absence of an understanding of treatment costs, clinicians and managers cannot know whether resources are being planned and used to best advantage, or whether they are already overstretched.

However, the initiative goes further than a system of costing and pricing services. Understanding the cost of a service is only part of the value-for-money equation. The quality of the service, treatment or episode must be established, so that the issue is not merely treatment X costs £Y, but treatment X to standard Z costs £Y.

The generation of the appropriate information alone does not ensure the effective management of resources. It has become clear from the experience at the six pilot sites that the management structure must be radically changed and devolved. This is a move away from historical management arrangements in which doctors, nurses and other health care professionals committed resources, but the actual control and authority to manage the overall budget rested with general managers. The Resource Management Initiative has seen the implementation of major organizational change to develop a situation in which those who take resource-consuming decisions, that is, the clinicians, are given the responsibility for managing those resources and the authority to alter allocation of their resources in the light of the appropriate information. This means that clinicians are not only entrusted with the responsibility for managing resources, but are given the authority to do so effectively.

Since the initial launch of the Resource Management Initiative, in 1986, currently some 260 acute hospital provider units have become involved in implementation.

Resource management and community care

The underlying philosophy of the Resource Management Initiative is that the delivery of care should be underpinned by effective management of resources. This necessitates informed decision-making based on accurate, timely and appropriate patient-based information. Evaluation of work already undertaken within the context of resource management highlights similarities between acute and community provider organizations.

Two pilot management budgeting projects within community health services were initiated in 1985 at Bromley and Worcester Health Authorities. Progress at these sites was reviewed by the Department of Health and reported in the Department of Health Notice, *Resource Management (Management Budgeting) in Health Authorities* (HN(86)34 1986). This outlined the strategy of the NHS Management Board to extend the approach to a small number of second generation sites, building on the work in the two original development sites.

Eleven second generation sites were established during 1987/8. They were joined by a twelfth site in 1989. Progress at these sites was reviewed by the NHS Management Executive (NHSME). Their report, *Resource Management in the Community Health Services* (1991) demonstrates the extent to which the resource management approach supports good practice in the community health service. As a result, the NHSME recommended the extension of resource management into the community health service.

Resource management within the community health services has the same objectives as resource management in other fields, i.e. it aims to achieve improvements in patient care through the better use of resources. The nature of community health services, however, is such that the major resource is staff time, predominantly community nursing, and generally using relatively autonomous individual professionals, although with an increasing emphasis on teamwork with a range of skills and grade mix. The service is delivered to a large extent in people's homes and this affects the pattern of resource use considerably. Resource management in the community will contribute to the improved use of information to ensure that staff spend as much time as possible with patients in targeted activities, within services that fit the needs of the local community. This has already been addressed in a number of community units to date.

Resource management and clinical services

Clinicians make important resource allocation decisions through the clinical and managerial judgements they make about the service they provide, the resources they choose to use and the way in which they manage them. Their involvement in management decision-making provides an opportunity to ensure that major resource allocation decisions are taken with clinical knowledge and experience. The clinical manager with responsibility for the budget has the authority to make resource allocation changes to adapt or improve the way that the service is provided. The devolved management structures provide the opportunity for collaboration on a multidisciplinary basis within a given specialty or locality. The development of more accurate information on the utilization of the clinical resource and the demand placed upon it by patients, relatives and other professionals enables clinicians to deploy resources to areas of greatest need. The devolution of managerial accountability to clinical managers has brought with it increasing pressures. Before the advent of clinical management teams, 'responsibility' for management issues was seen as a generalized obligation of professionals, that is, that they conducted their work in a manner consistent with agreed objectives, and with an authority granted to them through their professional hierarchy. Accountability is much more specific, it is the obligation to report on performance; it involves the keeping and disclosure of accurate records of the organization of clinical work, the care that patients receive and the resources used. To achieve this, information on professional and managerial action is paramount to enable the evaluation of service performance.

The Resource Management Initiative has become a supportive process, underpinning sound general management principles and the professional practice of health care delivery. Because of this it is concerned with all facets of the management and clinical process. Resource management comprises a multitude of interrelated and interdependent factors, cultural and attitudinal influences, organizational objectives and personal aspirations, professional and management values, technological developments and the effects of work organization; all of which can cause conflict or benefit to the organization depending on the way in which they are managed.

Effective resource management is a management process, not a discrete project or programme, which is how it has been widely viewed in the past. However, project management principles have been applied at the implementation phase of those funded projects to ensure that certain targets are achieved within specific timescales and budgets. Whilst the initiative was originally led by the Department of

Health, Regional Health Authorities have responsibility to support and facilitate the implementation programme within their regions.

For the purposes of this book, resource management will not be addressed in the context of the implementation programme but in its wider sense as a supportive process of health care delivery.

CONCLUSION

In the health care setting it is vital that decision making takes place as closely as possible to clinical services, to ensure that resources are where they are most needed and that patients' needs are being adequately met.

Resource management provides an opportunity to integrate quality of care thinking, dialogue and management. It also creates information and communication channels which cut across traditional management boundaries and professional tribalism, enabling the accountability for both the management of resources and the quality of care to be held at the nearest point of care delivery. Clear processes must be established for the planning, organization and control of resources to ensure that care services can respond quickly to the demands placed upon them.

Health care resources will always be finite, clinicians and managers need to develop stronger collaborative networks within the organization, and between other organizations and service users to develop partnerships that enhance current health care delivery, maximize resource use and enable local decisions to be taken with a broader understanding of health and health care delivery. The patient is now the primary focus for all activity, it is essential therefore to have comprehensive patient-based information to understand the resource consequences and care outcomes that are a result of professional or managerial interventions. But above all, the information must be of a high quality and managed in a way that provides benefit both to the individual patient and the service as a whole.

REFERENCES

HN(86)34 (1986) *Resource Management (Management Budgeting) in Health Authorities.* November.

NHSME (1991) *Resource Management in the Community Health Services.* London: Resource Management Unit, DoH.

HEALTH CARE ECONOMICS AND THE MANAGEMENT OF RESOURCES

2

Major debate inside and outside the health service will for the foreseeable future be focused on health care and resource issues. Little is known about the relationship and tensions associated between achieving the best outcome for the patient and the best value for money. Choosing among alternative forms of care when they differ in costs requires knowledge about the expected benefits, but also knowing when to provide more care and when to stop requires knowing something about the costs that inevitably must be paid and how those costs match the value of the health outcomes that are received in return.

CHAPTER AIMS

☐ To introduce the concept of health care economics

☐ To examine the structure of health care provision in terms of input, process and outcome

☐ **To introduce ethical and personal dilemmas in resource allocation**

☐ **To clarify the terms efficiency and effectiveness**

☐ **To examine the role of economic appraisal**

CONTEXT

Whilst the NHS is a non-profit organization, the introduction of major changes in the service make clear that a business-like culture is to be developed, with more attention focused on the effective management of resources and continual improvement in the quality of service provision. Effectiveness and value-for-money are now explicit objectives of health care management in the 1990s.

NHS activity continues to increase with 1991/92 showing a further 498,000 patients treated, a 7% increase on the previous year (with Trust hospitals treating 8% more patients). The acute sector alone handled 7.5 million completed consultant episodes against 7 million in 1990/91. Total gross spending on the NHS in 1991/92 was £26.9 billion, representing cash growth of 14%, and real growth of 6.5% (NHSME Annual Report 1991/92). Despite an overall increase in resources, many improvements to future services will need to be achieved within established expenditure levels.

Decisions within the health service about the development of services and use of resources have depended on a variety of factors, including perceived need, the volume of service, professional initiatives and political priorities, but have not previously incorporated systematic information about benefits to patients' health (Allen et al 1989). Rising costs and increased pressures on the resources available for health care in recent years have served to emphasize the need to incorporate economic analysis into choices in the health field (Drummond 1981).

The Resource Management Initiative was developed to provide a catalyst for such change. Resource management is a concept that brings together concerns about cost effective performance, with that of information provision and managerial participation and process. These concerns are encompassed within the general statement of principles in the Health Notice announcing the development of the Resource Management Initiative. The aim is to enable the NHS to give a better service to patients by helping clinicians and other managers to make better informed judgements about how the resources they control can be used to maximum effect. The programme's subsidiary objective was provision for clinicians of information which enables them to identify areas of waste and inefficiency, benefit from clinical group discussion and review, highlight areas which could most benefit from more resources, identify and expose the health care consequences of given financial policies and constraints, understand the comparative costs of future care options and hold informed debates about such options (HN(86)34 1986). This approach has embraced an economic discipline as a way of thinking and analysis for resource allocation decisions. A fundamental aspect of this approach is that health care professionals and general managers need to be aware that every health care intervention has clinical, social, and economic outcomes and that each of these factors must be considered and their implications understood when any treatment is decided upon.

Health economics is described as the overall health impact of the economy. Health care economics, on the other hand, describes the demand and supply of health care rather than health *per se*. The provision of health care is complex. It operates under economic, social, political and regulatory constraints in a professional and managerial environment. In considering how the resource management approach will assist in achieving the best outcome for the patient, and the best value for money within increasingly limited resources, it would be useful to contemplate the process of health care delivery.

The process of health care delivery

The operational structure of health care delivery is comprised of inputs, process, and output (see Figure 2.1). In terms of input, human, material and financial resources are available to support health care

Inputs

Financial resources
Material resources
Human resources
Information
Patients
Legal, fiscal and regulatory controls

Process

Organization structure
Model/protocol of care
Resource allocation and utilization
Flow of activities
Monitoring and control mechanisms

Output

Service throughput
  (number of discharges, number of deaths etc.)
Contracts delivery

Outcome

Appropriateness and acceptability
Degree of health gain
Patients satisfaction
Value

Figure 2.1: Health care organizations – operating structure

delivery. The amount or availability of these resources and the demand
for health care will continually change, and it is the responsibility of
the organization and its health care professionals to work together to

predict and plan for such changes and also to make informed judgements as to how those resources are to be allocated to meet demand. These inputs are combined in different ways to produce the processes of health care. These processes (a series of health care activities) describe the mechanisms necessary to ensure that the allocation and subsequent economic use of resources takes place. A process translates the inputs into outputs and outcomes. It is at this point that the issues of effectiveness and efficiency are mainly focused.

The outputs of health care delivery, although not obviously concerned with resources and their management, relate to the effectiveness and efficiency of their use. Efficiency may determine a measure of the output, for example, high throughput from shorter lengths of stay. Outcome is an evaluation of the output and indicates the effectiveness or otherwise of health care.

To assist clinicians and managers in understanding the process of health care delivery the essence of the resource management approach is to provide better information to support both clinicial and managerial decision-making. Improving health care information is focused at three very different levels. First, for the patient, this information must enable informed judgements to be made on the benefits or risks involved in choosing a certain treatment or course of action. Second, for the clinician, to advise patients and to record, monitor and evaluate their own practice; and third, for society as a whole to develop a responsible attitude to health, and to work with the health service to help to determine priorities for deploying whatever resources there are available for health care.

In determining the 'best outcome' for the patient and the 'best value for money' there is a need for clinicians to evaluate their activity, its cost to the patient and the service as a whole, the benefits that the intervention has provided, and the benefits that are lost by the utilization of the resources in a particular way. Given that resources are scarce if we decide to use them in one particular way, there is an opportunity foregone (described as an opportunity cost) to obtain the benefits of using these resources in some other way. The concept of 'opportunity cost' encourages us to place a monetary value on 'costs' which might not normally be seen as having pound signs in front of them, or indeed as costs at all (Mooney 1992).

The resource management approach supports and encourages the participation of health care professionals in management. It recognizes a need for all clinicians to become involved in strategic as well as operational management decision-making. It is the clinicians who are in the best position to know and plan the direction and speed at which their specialty and service is developing.

One of the main difficulties that face clinical managers is that of considering the service rather than individual patients. Clinicians are concerned with health and health care and yet traditionally they have focused much of their attention on disease because of the view that eliminating disease contributes to improving health. Maxwell (1985) indicated that physicians had a duty to study and take account of the needs of the community as a whole, since the concept of the patient presenting as the only patient that matters is too narrow; to use resources with parsimony, since they are limited and good medicine does not have to be extravagant; to question constantly what is good in patient care and what is not, using sound scientific methods to differentiate between the two; to help every patient and every community to help themselves as far as possible; to create elbow room for continuing change in clinical practice and to contribute imaginatively and unselfishly to a clear definition of where the institution or service is heading and why. Maxwell also emphasized that while we must accept the reality of finite resource limits, we must also test them, and try to use the money available more flexibly.

Resource management and ethical considerations

There will certainly be ethical and personal dilemmas in considering the allocation of resources for patient care. Mooney (1992) identifies three principal theories of ethics: the ethics of virtue, of duty and of the common good. The first two are essentially individualistic ethics and the last a social ethic. Medical ethics deals in the main with the theories of virtue and duty, but the nature of contemporary medicine and health service management philosophy increasingly demands that these be complemented by the third theory – the common good. Constructive dialogue between such forums as Regional Medical Committees, Purchasing Authorities and Public Health specialists will serve to develop a more realistic appraisal of service development, consumer need and the common good. At a macro level (the Department of Health, the Regional Health Authorities and the District Health Authorities) the emphasis of resource allocation and management will increasingly be driven through a social ethical base primarily because of the new public health philosophy. However, at a micro level (the doctor and patient) consideration must be given to the individual ethical base where conflicts will undoubtedly arise if resources are diverted away from the individual to serve the common good.

The resource management approach serves to highlight the ethical considerations that must be made when allocating resources to one group rather than another, or to one intervention rather than another. Judgements about what is ethical will necessitate a professional view supported by comprehensive audit information and clinical group discussion. There can be no real debate about identifying and choosing between resource allocation priorities until more is known about the costs and benefits of many existing clinical practices. Until such robust information is available it will be extremely difficult to address the more sensitive task of choosing between them. Ethical considerations until that time will be governed by medical rather than social ethics. The extent to which individual clinicians allow resource constraints to influence their behaviour will remain a matter for individual clinical judgement. A fundamental role of economic analysis is to identify the implications of alternative ways of responding to that dilemma.

Effectiveness and efficiency

In considering outcome and its effectiveness, one must appraise the benefits or harm that the patient is exposed to through health care intervention. Benefits may be categorized as a reduction in costs; changes in health state, e.g. reduction of distress, increase in life expectancy, and an increase in quality of life; and changes in productive output, e.g. ability to gain employment. The changes in health status and changes in productive output are largely determined by clinical measurement. In health service management costs have traditionally be seen as a cost to the service itself. Whilst it is accepted that many health care interventions can bring about resource changes in other sectors of the economy, for example the local authority, there is little acknowledgement given to the cost implications to patients and their families. The patient and family consume their own personal resources (money and time). This resource use does not result in health service expenditure and so is easily discounted, but in economic terms these changes represent very real costs to the community. The scale of these costs must not be underestimated, the 1985 OPCS survey suggested that there were approximately 6 million carers in Great Britain, of whom about a quarter were spending 20 or more hours a week in caring. Looking after a dependent person imposes several costs, in particular loss of income, but also personal stress and illness from continual caring (Audit Commission 1992). From a clinical perspective these are hidden and in the main unappreciated costs which will only be highlighted by using economic analysis techniques.

An important aspect of outcome is measuring the effectiveness or otherwise of clinical intervention and management practice. Effectiveness is concerned with 'doing the right things', and relates to output (the end result) as well as the health outcome (assessment of the extent to which benefit has been achieved and attributing that benefit to the health care intervention). Doing the right thing means identifying the options, estimating the outcomes of each option, and choosing or helping the patient to choose the best option. Effectiveness is a measure of how successfully or otherwise activities are being carried out. Whilst the measurement of output can be quantified, e.g. number of discharges, number of theatre cases etc., the measurement of outcome is qualitative and therefore more difficult to determine. Some measures include mortality, readmission rates, iatrogenic admissions, post-operative complications, changes in health status, altered life expectancy, patient satisfaction etc. Outcomes are in many instances intangible or may need to be measured over long periods of time, for example in relation to the measurement of health gain where long periods of rehabilitation are necessary before measurement of recovery can take place. In resource allocation decision-making, clinical information and appraisal can indicate some of the desirable and undesirable effects of clinical intervention, but unless this is complemented by an analysis of resource costs it cannot advise the clinician or manager of the benefits foregone.

Efficiency is concerned with 'doing things right', that is, how we do things – ensuring maximum resource use (no matter how small an allocation), to provide maximum benefit to the patient. Doing the wrong things less expensively becomes costly. Doing things right first time, every time, supports the quality manager's maxim 'quality costs less'. Efficient care is the method of achieving a stated level of care at the lowest cost. It is important to note at this stage that the cheapest activity is not necessarily the most efficient, as both the quality and quantity of activity must be considered. Energies must be focused on minimizing costs and maximizing benefits.

Although efficiency intentions are important in decision-making, they cannot reveal the complete picture, which is essential in health care delivery. For example, there is no useful purpose in deploying staff efficiently if patient care is not effectively provided. The effectiveness of a service must be determined by both the professionals providing the service and the users of the service to establish whether or not it can be described as effective. Effectiveness, therefore, considers the characteristics of the outcome as well as the efficiency of its delivery (see Figures 2.2 and 2.3).

An effective and efficient service will only be achieved through well informed planning and responsive management; and the development of structures and processes which support the balance of resource input and utilization to provide effective health care. Monitoring the input of resources and the process of their utilization provides limited information to determine the outcome that will be achieved for the

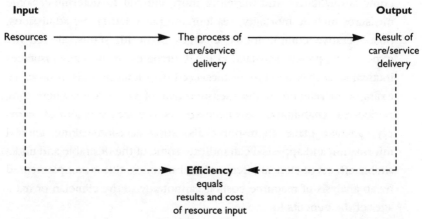

Figure 2.2: Operational efficiency. Adapted from Cooke and Slack (1984)

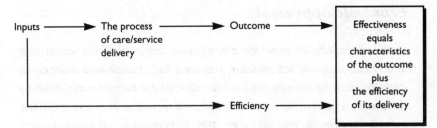

Figure 2.3: Efficiency and effectiveness of service delivery. Adapted from Cooke and Slack (1984)

given input. Without a wider use of economics in health care inefficiencies will abound and decisions will be made less explicitly and hence less rationally than is desirable: we will go on spending large sums to save life in one way when similar lives in greater numbers could be saved in another way (Mooney 1992). Such inefficiency is unethical and highlights the value of analysing both the costs and benefits of alternative patterns of care, because only with such analysis can the 'best buy' be identified and adopted (Maynard 1985). Cochrane (1971), a well-respected physician whose renowned book *Effectiveness and Efficiency* focused on the need for more evaluative work of clinical practice to determine clinical effectiveness and control efficiency showed that the potential conflicts between the more conservative attitudes to clinical freedom and the pursuit of efficiency need to be resolved.

From an economic standpoint, achieving value for money must also consider the sensitive and challenging issue of rationing health care. The BMA in its discussion document *Leading for Health* (1991) identified that rationing was already a reality in the health service. The report states that there is a strong argument that a substantial increase in funding would largely resolve the problem of rationing, although some of those consulted thought that this would only be a temporary solution. Most agreed that the NHS and community care services could never meet all patient needs and expectations. There thus seems to be a clear need to prioritize and ration services, where resources are finite their scarcity makes choice inevitable. Rationing, however, inevitably raises ethical questions. Sometimes these concern choices that must be made between individual patients, at other times the choices are between preventive or curative health care programmes.

Economic appraisal

Economic appraisal provides a systematic framework for identifying and organizing the information required for clinical and managerial decision-making. Its aim is to ensure that all the factors surrounding a decision are taken into account and, where possible, quantified and valued (Ludbrook and Mooney 1984). Economic appraisal cannot replace decision-making and value judgements, it is a supportive process, based on facts to ensure that as much benefit as possible is obtained from the resources devoted to health care. Since economic appraisal will rely partly on clinical appraisal through audit for the assessment of changes in health status, it is important to note that economic appraisal is only as complete and factual as the clinical appraisal with which it is integrated.

Economic appraisal is likely to be useful where large amounts of limited resources are involved; where responsibility for resources is uncoordinated and fragmented; and where there exist alternatives for resource use; and where different benefits and costs can be identified. Given that there is always more than one course of action, the existence of choices therefore gives the scope for appraisal. Whilst cost containment and efficiency are important considerations in the management of resources, they cannot and must not be divorced from quality of care issues.

CONCLUSION

The finite resource of the NHS as in healthcare management worldwide, charges managers with the task of achieving value i.e. to concern themselves with determining efficiency, effectiveness and value priorities. Achieving value for money is concerned with determining efficiency, effectiveness and value.

All of us commit ourselves to certain value judgements unknowingly. It is important to note that the value placed on various outcomes by patients may differ from those placed on them by professionals. 'Consumer sovereignty' suggests that it is the consumer's values which are the right ones in judging the benefits of health programmes, this however is not so simple and is made more complex by the individual's lack of knowledge and lack of rationality. Clinicians need to be particularly sensitive to the patient's values if they are to act in the patient's interest. Because of the subjectivity of value judgements, the issues surrounding valuation in health care are fraught with difficulty. Mooney (1985) stated that one of the most fundamental questions underlying the stresses, strains and conflicts over the health service is not related to whether we can place a money value on human life. There is no debate here. We do. The question is rather: whose values are appropriate?

ACTION GUIDELINES

The following guidelines will help you identify the significant areas for action in your clinical service:

1 What are the key objectives set out in the business plan of your organization?

2 List five efficiency initiatives which could be or have been introduced in your organization.

3 In what way is the demand for your particular service changing?

4 What are the main influences which affect demand for your service?

5 How do you evaluate the outcome of your care?

6 Discuss with colleagues the dilemmas faced by yourselves as clinicians because of resource constraints.

REFERENCES

Allen D, Lee R and Lowson K (1989) The use of QALYs in health service planning *International Journal of Health Planning and Management*, **4**; 261–273.

Audit Commission (1992) *The Community Revolution: Personal Social Services and Community Care*. London: HMSO.

BMA (1991) *Leading for Health: A BMA Agenda for Health*. London.

Cochrane A L (1971) *Effectiveness and Efficiency: Random Reflections on Health Services*. Nuffield Provincial Hospitals Trust.

Cooke S and Slack N (1984) *Making Management Decisions*. London: Prentice Hall.

Drummond M (1981) Economic appraisal in health care *Hospital and Health Service Review*, **Oct**: 277–281.

HN(86)34 (1986) *Resource Management (Management Budgeting) in Health Authorities*. November.

Ludbrook A and Mooney G (1984) *Economic Appraisal in the NHS: Problems and Challenges*. Northern Health Economics, Health Economics Research Unit, University of Aberdeen.

Maxwell RJ (1985) Resource constraints and the quality of care *The Lancet*. 26 October.

Maynard A (1985) In search of efficiency *Health and Social Service Journal*, 18 July.

Mooney G (1985) Valuing human life in health service policy *Nuffield/York Portfolios* **3**.

Mooney G (1992) *Economics, Medicine and Health Care*, 2nd Edn. London: Harvester Wheatsheaf.

NHS (1991–1992) *Annual Report*. London: HMSO.

OPCS (1985) *Informal Carers*: Supplement to the General Household Survey 1985. London: HMSO.

FURTHER READING

☐ Bowling A (1991) *Measuring Health*. Buckingham: Open University Press.

☐ Cochrane A L (1971) *Effectiveness and Efficiency: Random Reflections on Health Services*. Nuffield Provincial Hospitals Trust.

☐ Ludbrook A and Mooney G (1984) *Economic Appraisal in the NHS: Problems and Challenges*. Northern Health Economics, Health Economics Research Unit, University of Aberdeen.

☐ Mooney G (1986) *Economics, Medicine and Health Care*. London: Harvester Wheatsheaf.

INFORMATION MANAGEMENT

3

The **NHS** is undergoing a revolution in the management and use of information. Managers and clinicians need reliable information more quickly than ever to make decisions and to organize work within budget and under other constraints. Millions of pounds are being spent on computer hardware and software to improve information systems. Much of this will be wasted if people do not learn to manage and use information.

CHAPTER AIMS

☐ To explore the concept of information

☐ To identify the increasing role of information in decision-making

☐ To discuss the information needs of clinicians

☐ To discuss the use of information technology as an aid to managers

☐ To consider the potential benefits of information management and technology

CONTEXT

Clinicians need credible information to support meaningful dialogue with other professionals and general managers when setting resource priorities. Where real commitment to the involvement of professionals in the management process takes place, clinical managers will have the managerial authority to influence both strategic and operational decisions. Decision-making in the 1990s will be increasingly information based.

In 1863 Florence Nightingale observed:

> In attempting to arrive at the truth I have applied everywhere for information but in scarcely an instance have I been able to obtain hospital records fit for any purpose of comparison. If they could be obtained they would enable us to decide many other questions besides the one alluded to. They would show subscribers how their money was being spent, what amount of good was really being done with it or whether the money was not doing mischief rather than good
>
> (Nightingale 1863)

This statement supports present day thinking in relation to quality and resource management issues in health care. Progress to establish a comprehensive information base has been and will continue to be slow, particularly if widespread variation in practice and professional opinion continues.

Information

Information is a message, it is composed of data, which can be described as the raw material from which the information is extracted and analysed, and then supplied in a suitable form for a specific purpose, for example, decision material and intelligence material (research or background data). Data requires processing to become information and in the same way, information requires processing to become meaningful and useful. Information provides a powerful tool to analyse a situation, and enable the user to form an opinion and ultimately support the decision process.

Information is used to support many professional and managerial functions:

- ☐ Planning – the bringing together of information in order to formulate strategic and operational plans.

- ☐ Control – information is essential to monitor the work of the organization and evaluate its efficiency and effectiveness.

- ☐ Research and audit – information to identify wide variations in practice and to measure the effectiveness or otherwise of clinical interventions, analysis into the content and delivery of health care is necessary.

- ☐ Decision making – information will be reviewed by the professional/manager and choices made on the basis of the information received.

- ☐ Intelligence gathering – this is a necessary technique in determining a whole range of information related to the internal and external environment, for example, market research, patient satisfaction, and audit.

Characteristics of information

The user must be aware of the comprehensiveness and validity of the information. Data can easily be distorted and corrupted, understanding its source and determining its quality is a necessary task before it can be put to good use. Information, it should always be remembered, is rarely perfect.

DEGREE OF DETAIL

As more information is obtained its value may diminish as the volume increases and it can soon become unmanageable or confusing to the user. It is essential therefore to establish through discussion with information users the level of detail needed to support a given task or decision. This should of course be reviewed regularly and adjusted as necessary; as the service changes so will information requirements. It is always important to establish the relevance, adequacy and necessity of the information received.

SOURCE

The source of the data will affect the confidence a professional or manager has in the information presented. There is a need to be reassured through constant review that the data and its collection is credible, otherwise the information will not be used and the whole process of collection and analysis becomes a wasteful and costly exercise.

RELIABILITY AND VALIDITY

Reliability is the extent to which the same data will consistently provide the same results. Validity is essential for drawing conclusions and is the extent to which a particular measure reflects what it is supposed to measure. An instrument can be reliable but not valid for its intended purpose (Holland 1983).

USEFULNESS

Collection and analysis of data must be determined by the users, otherwise the information will have no clinical or managerial value. The information should be presented in a form which enables it to be used directly. Information is of no value itself and is important only because of the uses to which it is put. Information that has a multiple purpose, for example, for use by nurses, other professionals and managers, will prove to be a cost effective option.

AGE

Information becomes dated immediately after it is produced, the age of the information must always be considered in relation to its usefulness.

TIMELINESS

Timeliness is the time between the data being collected, analysed and returned to the user as usable information. If there is a long time lag then the information loses its credibility as events or decisions may already have taken place. It is clearly important that the information must be available when the decision has to be made.

COST

The information should not cost more to obtain than the benefit its knowledge produces. The greater the accuracy and volume of the information, the greater its cost; this is largely due to the technology necessary and the time taken for the collection and analysis of the data.

Information Requirements

One of the most necessary and sometimes the most difficult task facing clinicians and managers is the correct identification of information requirements. It is important to be able to 'track' all activity, that is, from the inputs to the service, how they are utilized, and what was achieved, to provide a complete picture (see Figure 3.1).

DETERMINING NEEDS AND DEMANDS

The need for health care can be regarded as the sum of needs of individuals in the community or as the difference between actual and optimum levels of health without consideration of the availability of services. Information on the population's health care demands (what people ask for) and needs (what people could benefit from) is essential to ensure that the supply of services available is targeted to those areas of need, and that demands, in so far as is possible, are also met. Health authorities, purchasing health care on behalf of their resident popu-

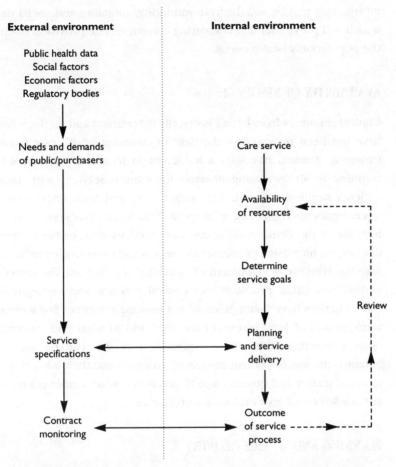

External environment

Public health data
Social factors
Economic factors
Regulatory bodies

Needs and demands
of public/purchasers

Service
specifications

Contract
monitoring

Internal environment

Care service

Availability
of resources

Determine
service goals

Planning
and service
delivery

Outcome
of service
process

Review

Figure 3.1: Information sources and flow in relation to a provider unit

lation, will be responsible for the assessment of health care needs. The 'need' identified by the health authority will depend on how many people have a particular problem, that is, the number becoming ill each year (incidence) and number remaining ill at any one time (prevalence). Purchasers of health care are actively seeking a perspective of what services they might purchase in the future by obtaining the views of the local population, general practitioners and other providers of care; and comparing the provision of health care locally with that in other Health Authorities and Family Health Service Authorities. This information will be sought from morbidity, mortality and social data which will prove useful in comparing current service provision against the population's health needs.

AVAILABILITY OF RESOURCES

Clinical resources have been historically determined and on the whole have not been reviewed in the light of changing health care needs. Changing demand has seen a reduction in length of hospital stay, resulting in an increasing demand for clinical services with more patients needing concentrated skilled care, and with fewer convalescent patients remaining in hospital. This in turn has resulted in an increase in the demand on community services from earlier hospital discharges. Increasing consumer awareness and participation in health care has seen the development of individualized care and the removal of task orientated practices. For clinical practice and management these changes have taken place within existing resources but without a reappraisal of how resources are used and to what end. Accurate clinical information provides a valuable tool that can be used to enhance the use of present resources, to determine their adequacy in terms of quality and quantity and to determine what further resources are needed to achieve health care objectives.

PLANNING AND SERVICE DELIVERY

All plans should be based on clearly defined objectives and use made of all available information. Strategic planning, for example, requires information on manpower requirements to meet the organization's objectives whilst the process of service delivery will involve the operational planning of how the strategically identified manpower resources will be used to help meet these objectives in delivering health care on a day-to-day basis.

OUTCOMES OF SERVICE DELIVERY

Outcome indicates the effectiveness or otherwise of health care. It is the essential measurement of output, and information is the evaluation tool.

Information and audit

There is a strong interest now being shown by the Royal Colleges in developing audit and the very practical advice and help becoming available to support clinical staff in this area demonstrates the way forward. The impact of individual staff and their decisions on the care of the patient means that each person involved in care delivery needs to understand their duty and responsibilities as well as their professional commitment towards maintaining quality care. In consideration of this, thought needs to be given to the role of all clinicians and non-clinical staff whose work is supportive to the care of the patient.

There is clearly a need therefore to develop audit within each professional group, but more importantly the interface between the different clinical groups needs to be examined with the further development of clinical audit systems. Discussions between nursing and medical staff, for example, have revealed a lack of awareness and understanding of the totality of care being delivered. Even in units where there are well formulated protocols which are well understood by all clinical professionals the whole course of treatment still relies on the co-operation and co-working of non-clinical professionals.

It should be remembered that audit is not a new idea or activity. The many and varied reasons for examining and evaluating clinical practice have long inspired practitioners to undertake local studies, develop methods for audit, and to set up major reviews of practice. The purpose of audit is to improve the quality of care that health care professionals provide for their patients by evaluating the effectiveness of current practice; improving practice both individually and within departments; enhancing professional development and education and evaluating effectiveness and efficiency of resource use. With the audit process still in its infancy it will take several years before formal systems are fully developed; however, the critical element of all audit systems, from the most primitive to the most sophisticated, is that they should alter clinical practice for the better. The audit process and the resource management approach share the goals of effectiveness and efficiency with the patient as the focus for all activity.

Audit supports management by the generation of information which should underpin decisions in planning and evaluating service provision. Audit information will guide changes in professional practice.

The link between effective resource management and quality is inextricably bound by the knowledge that this information will provide.

Information management and technology

It cannot be over emphasized that health care resources will always be finite, increasing pressure is being placed on clinicians and managers to develop robust practices that enhance current health care delivery, maximize resource use and enable local decisions to be taken with a broader understanding of health and health care delivery. With the patient being the primary focus for clinical and managerial activity, the development of comprehensive patient-based information is essential to facilitate a better understanding of the resource consequences and care outcomes that are a result of professional or managerial inter-ventions. This information must be of a high quality and managed in a way that provides benefit both to the individual patient and the service as a whole. Information is the lifeblood of the NHS:

> There can be no doubt that information and information technology will have a major role to play in the post review NHS. To reap all the considerable benefits of the changes, the NHS will need to make progress in such matters as the letting and management of contracts and the definition and measurement of quality of care, as well as the management of resources. To do all this, health care organisations will need improved information systems and the appropriate infor-mation technology to support them.
>
> (Freeman 1990)

Information technology is a technology that dramatically increases the ability to record, store, analyse and transmit information in ways that permit flexibility, accuracy, immediacy, geographic independence, volume, and complexity (Zuboff 1989). The NHS generates vast amounts of data which is stored either as an indication of what is currently happening in the organization, or as a past record of what has happened. The difficulties the service has experienced have been the retrieval and assimilation of this data into comprehensive and useful information. Data is not information. Information is not meaning. Just as data requires processing to become informational, so information requires processing to become meaningful (Levitt 1990). Information technology provides the vehicle for transferring data into a form that with a manager's skill can become informational.

Information technology can improve the performance of health care organizations in many ways, both directly and indirectly; directly, through improving the clinical and managerial database to enhance decision-making, and indirectly, by the subsequent use of the data to provide meaningful information to clinicians and managers to inform management and clinical practice with the overriding objective of enhancing service delivery. It provides new channels of information and improves the quality of the information available to the clinician or manager by reducing the problems of inaccuracy, incompleteness, unavailability of data, written errors and delays that occur in manual information systems. As a by-product of the technology, information will be produced which if used effectively will create a broad view of the organization's operations by providing a deeper level of transparency to activities that had previously been difficult to monitor and evaluate.

The implementation of information technology within the clinical environment is a relatively new development, and because of this can be fascinating in its own right. The dangers this brings are twofold, first, that the computer becomes the focus for care assessment and evaluation rather than the patient, and second, that there is an unshakable belief that whatever information the computer provides is correct. It must be recognized that technology has limitations and these must not be overlooked: it lacks commonsense, instinct, experience, and sensitivity. The technology is a tool and must remain so, it should not be used simply because it is there. The machine itself cannot tell the user for what purpose it should be used or how problems are to be solved.

As implementation is planned and carried out, the organization has a responsibility to ensure that these opportunities are grasped and benefits for the patients, staff and organization realized. A benefits identification and realization programme must be undertaken prior to system selection to establish the potential benefits information technology would provide the organization, its staff and the patient, and whether the cost of implementing and maintaining such a system is justified. As implementation progresses it is also important to monitor if benefits are being realized, so that early intervention and support is accessible as difficulties arise.

The problems in implementing information technology will also have been identified prior to system selection and used as part of the selection process, whilst these will be anticipated problems, there will arise during implementation a substantial number of problems that need to be managed quickly and effectively. Where new technology is being implemented or current technology developed, a structured management framework is essential to ensure that all possible benefit is realized in as short a time as possible, with the least disruption to the organization. 'Project management' is one such methodology. Chapter 6 is dedicated to the principles of project management.

The implementation of information technology should recognize the concerns and aspirations of the individuals who will work with it. Considerable energy therefore needs to be invested in creating the cultural changes necessary before and during the introduction of technology, if full ownership and so the benefits of information technology are to be achieved. Senior care staff will have completed their formal education before computers became widespread. There is likely to be considerable fear of the machines and a lack of appreciation of the variety of functions available. There are at least three levels of staff who will need education and training to realize any major benefits from such an investment. These are senior managers who will make investment decisions and manage the implementation; senior care staff, such as doctors, nurses and other health care professionals, who will use computers in their daily work to access information and analyse data for day-to-day business; and clerical and junior care staff who will enter data into the computer and assure its accuracy and completeness (Ledwith 1991). The time to be invested in the necessary training and education to prepare staff to use computers cannot be overestimated, the cost of this training must be assessed and adequate investment made. The emphasis on using information for clinical and managerial decision-making has developed rapidly in the NHS over the last few years; it is important therefore that staff are skilled in the analysis, presentation and management of data to ensure that the information can be used to ensure that the benefits of the system are realized. Training and development is paramount to ensure that staff are informed, involved and supported.

At an operational level, the successful implementation of information technology is dependent on the following factors:

☐ involvement of key personnel at all key stages of the selection and implementation of the technology;

☐ the chosen technology should be able to meet all the essential information requirements identified by the organization;

☐ sensitive guidance and change management takes place during the implementation stage;

☐ a comprehensive education and training programme is provided;

☐ speedy and reliable access to system maintenance is made available, for example, 'Help Desk' facilities;

☐ the system design should be flexible in approach and capable of expansion as technology, practice and information requirements change.

At the individual manager level, management is becoming increasingly 'information intensive'. The handling of information of all types and its integration into effective information systems and services is increasingly seen as essential if organizations are to operate effectively in times of technological and environmental change (Broadbent 1991)

There is now a need for all managers to have a much better grasp of the impact of information technology and information, just as there is a need for information managers and specialists to understand the requirements of the 'business' and 'care' aspects of the health care organization in which they work.

CONCLUSION

Through information, the intellectual foundation of health care is being challenged, the challenge is justified by a real concern for the quality, effectiveness, efficiency and efficacy of current health care delivery.

Information provides a powerful tool to analyse a situation, and enables the user to form an opinion and ultimately support the decision process. Decision-making in the 1990s will be increasingly information-based with clinical as well as general managers needing credible information to influence both strategic and operational management.

Clinical managers must be aware of the comprehensiveness and validity of the information they use. Distorted or corrupted data will undermine and discredit management decisions. Information, it should always be remembered, is rarely perfect.

Information technology has become fundamental in supporting the managerial routines such as administrative tasks and the day-to-day operations of health care organizations. Although use of technology itself can be time consuming, it can in a wider context save time, for example, by communicating information quickly throughout the organization which may take hours or weeks using manual methods. Historically senior managers 'controlled' the information, now with clinicians gaining access to their own information, this has enabled them to derive some independence as managers creating greater initiative in clinical and managerial decision-making.

Ultimately, the introduction of technology will facilitate the development of a comprehensive patient database. This information will enable clinicians and managers to capture and compare the contribution made by each professional for each patient/patient group; it will describe the resources needed to treat a particular patient group in relation to appropriateness, quality and cost; it will provide a focus for the monitoring and evaluation of treatment outcomes, and it will provide a catalyst for research and development to facilitate the development of treatment protocols and standards.

ACTION GUIDELINES

The following guidelines will help you identify the significant areas for action relating to information and its management in supporting your clinical and managerial decision-making:

1 What information do you need in order to deliver clinical care to your patients/clients?

2 What managerial information do you need to manage your part of the service?

3 What aspect(s) of your information requirement is mandatory?

4 Discuss with colleagues the actual and potential uses of information technology in your area

5 How could you conduct an audit in your own area of work?

REFERENCES

Broadbent M (1991) Information management: strategies and alliances *Aslib Proceedings*: **43** (1) January.

Freeman R (1990) Information the lifeblood of the NHS *Health Service Journal*, March.

Holland W (1983) *Evaluation of Health Care*. Oxford: OUP.

Ledwith F (1991) Know I.T., Know NHS *British Journal of Healthcare Computing*, September.

Levitt T (1990) The thinking manager *Health Management Quarterly*: **2**.

Nightingale F (1863) *Notes on Hospitals* (3rd edn). London: Langman.

Zuboff S (1989) *In the Age of the Smart Machine*. New York: Basic Books Inc.

FURTHER READING

☐ Regional Consortium (Five Regions) (1991) *Using Information in Managing the Nursing Resource, A Learning Programme*. Macclesfield, Cheshire: Greenhalgh & Co. Ltd.

☐ Zuboff S (1989) *In the Age of the Smart Machine*. London: Heinemann.

THE HUMAN RESOURCE

4

It is now increasingly accepted that the effectiveness of service organizations are largely dependent upon the quality of their people. In the NHS, the traditional attitude to manpower has been one of a cost to the service, but with recent reforms and the growing need for all parts of the service to become consumer responsive, a growing realization that staff are a valuable investment has begun to take place.

CHAPTER AIMS

☐   To highlight the importance of considering people as individuals as well as meeting service needs and patient demand

☐   To set in context the issues of manpower planning

CONTEXT

Drucker says of the human resource, that the whole man is, of all resources entrusted to man, the most productive, the most versatile, and the most resourceful (Drucker 1989). With present and anticipated (mid 1990s) skills shortages great care must now be taken to retain and develop health care professionals working within the organization. The development of an innovative, empowered, enthusiastic and skilled workforce should be a prime objective for all clinical and general managers. Professionals in their efforts to protect their 'professionalism' need to be particularly careful not to distance themselves from the reality of changing service provision. Education and training must become more sensitive to supporting both the practitioner and management roles of clinicians in a continually changing work environment, without compromising professional values and beliefs, but with a determination to move forward and develop the health care professionals' contribution to present health care thinking and delivery. Opportunities to prepare staff for change have been sadly missed by the professions and general management – it is the operational manager who must now take a leading role in managing the staff they are responsible for. Much of managing the human resource is about managing people at work, understanding their needs, supporting them to use the skills they have, and maximizing their potential.

Supply and demand

Health care provision is labour intensive, and to ensure that an adequate supply of staff is available it is necessary to determine the demand for the clinical workforce and to plan to make certain that the demand is met. To inform planning, there needs to be an understanding of the work that will be generated by consumers, purchasers and colleagues (the work practices of others can influence an increase/decrease in workload), along with an understanding of manpower availability (see Figure 4.1). Strategic planning aims to identify the demand for and the supply of manpower in the future so that the right amount of skills can be available when necessary. Strategic decisions related to manpower supply must always be rationalized to meet

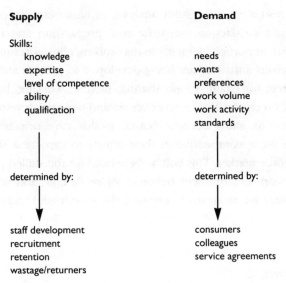

Supply	Demand
Skills:	
knowledge	needs
expertise	wants
level of competence	preferences
ability	work volume
qualification	work activity
	standards
determined by:	determined by:
staff development	consumers
recruitment	colleagues
retention	service agreements
wastage/returners	

Figure 4.1: Features of supply and demand

demand (market forces), for example, training for training's sake is wasteful and demoralizing for new qualifiers who cannot obtain jobs. Professionals have an obligation to ensure that the newly qualified are employable, but equally, that they are employed. Strategic planning has needed to be particularly sensitive to demographic changes and the subsequent difficulties in recruitment, because of this and anticipated short falls in skills, manpower planning has developed a much wider perspective to involve not only the acquisition of new skills but also the utilization, development and retention of current skills. Recruitment, retention and return to work strategies were until recently developed at district level, but now as provider units develop local strategies a bottom-up approach using skills audit, activity and trends analysis ensures that this process is now provider led.

There are a range of methodologies and techniques available to assist workforce planners in forecasting the planning and acquisition of resources, for example, personnel assessment methods and statistical forecasting methods. Analysis of demographic changes, unemployment trends and labour market competition from other service sectors are essential to understand why and when the shortfalls will take place. A robust strategy can then be developed to counteract the forecasted shortfall in supply. To ensure the effective deployment of existing human resources, work study analysis, an understanding of staff motivation and satisfaction, adequate role preparation and realistic job design are important elements in maximizing clinical resources.

Numerous initiatives are being developed to provide stability to the workforce, for example, job sharing, flexible working, back-to-work courses, crèche facilities, career breaks and personal development programmes. As skills become scarce health care organizations will become more competitive in their efforts to capture a share of the labour force market. This will be beneficial for the skilled professional as the work environment becomes more flexible and staff benefits more attractive as means to improve the recruitment and retention of staff.

Skill mix

Skill mix has emerged as a prominent issue in health care provision, at a time when new demands and priorities are identified within the service which both general managers and the professions need to address. Skill mix is a highly complex issue, with many interrelated and interdependent factors. Skill mix is inseparable from the job to be done, the number and type of skills necessary to do it and the needs and aspirations of those carrying out the work. The goal is to achieve locally (at care level) a mix of staff (professional and others), to provide high quality, cost effective care that meets the standards and goals of the organization (ward, directorate, locality or unit) and to meet the needs and expectations of those receiving and giving care. The achievement of an effective, efficient and appropriate skill mix has remained not surprisingly, elusive to many.

There are now increasing pressures for general managers and health care professionals to address this issue urgently. Skilled professional time is a crucial but expensive investment and as manpower is one of the most costly items of any provider unit's budget, understandably focus is being placed on its use and effectiveness as a service. General management pressures include ensuring value for money, the development of a good quality, consumer responsive service and ensuring that contractual agreements are met. As clinical accountability for resource management develops, the responsibility for determining optimal skill mix is shifting from general management to clinical managers. The professional's willingness to address this issue has been influenced by a number of factors:

☐ increasing demand on professional services with shorter lengths of patient stay, resulting in increased patient activity and an overall higher patient dependency;

☐ changing work organization and professional practices, particularly medical practice, which will affect the number and type of skills required;

☐ the need for a more flexible workforce, firstly for strategic planning, to take into consideration demographic changes and the difficulties in recruitment that this will bring; including the need to reduce a transient workforce through positive recruitment, retention and return to work strategies. Second, for operational planning to ensure the effective deployment and subsequent utilization of the clinical resource;

☐ increasing accountability for budgetary control has encouraged a more formal review of vacant posts, where traditionally like would have been replaced with like. Now, clinical managers are beginning to look at what funds they have, what skills they need to achieve a given standard of care, and the most cost effective options for obtaining those skills.

WHAT IS SKILL?

Skill is difficult to define. The *Oxford English Dictionary* defines skill as an expertness, a practised ability. Skill may be separated into two components, mental skill (abilities required for social interaction, calculation etc.) and action skill (abilities required for activity). Management theorists describe skill in the context of work productivity, categorizing skill into four components of technical, human, conceptual and design skills (see Table 4.1). These skills categorizations are clearly transposable to health care professionals and their work. Technical skill identifies the practitioner's knowledge of and proficiency in

Table 4.1: Skill categories

Skill category	Definition
Technical	Knowledge and proficiency in activity
Human	Ability to work with people, to communicate and interact with others
Conceptual	Ability to understand the wider picture
Design	Ability to work out a practical, logical solution to a problem

activities involving methods, processes, and procedures. Human skill identifies the practitioner's ability to work with people, to communicate effectively, and to function in a team and relate comfortably with other team members. It is particularly the human skills that reflect the traditional role of health care professionals, that is the caring for others and the development of the practitioner/patient relationship. Conceptual skill identifies the practitioner's ability to see the 'big picture', for example, to understand health in its wider context of physical, mental, and social well-being rather than to continue to perpetuate a disease focus and to understand that the clinical service is but one part of a whole series of support processes that the patient may need. Conceptual skill also encompasses a recognition of significant elements in a situation and to understand the relationships among the elements, for example, to understand that what might be beneficial for the professional may not be beneficial to the patient or the organization, and being able to work towards reconciling those differences. Design skill identifies the practitioner's ability to work out a practical, logical solution to a problem in a way that will enhance the situation. This is of particular importance as management responsibilities are devolved and where increasingly, judgements relating to the feasibility, effectiveness and efficacy of service provision have to be made.

Health care professionals are often unaware of the diversity and flexibility of their skills, and clinical managers have in many instances, either through ignorance or self interest, restricted skills development in their staff. Because of this many practitioners have been confined to what some perceive as the 'natural' role of their own profession, which in turn has resulted in their becoming trapped in narrow, stereotyped roles rather than being able to expand their personal and professional development more creatively.

It is important at this stage to make it clear that skill does not necessarily equate with grade or qualification. Practitioners have many skills but it is the identification of the appropriate skills necessary to meet specific demands at the required quality, that is needed to determine the right skill mix. The clinical team is a mixed workforce consisting of professional staff, learners, and support staff with some training, all of whom require varying degrees of supervision.

Skill mix can be described as the necessary proportion of staff, qualifications, levels of competence, abilities, knowledge and expertise, to achieve an agreed standard of care for a given level of demand. A skill mix, therefore, consists of more than one person and possibly a group of people, working and interacting together, with common goals. The structure (leadership and organization), composition (professional and non-professional, skills, expertise, specialist knowledge) and size of the group will depend largely on the nature of the work. Other factors are supply, traditional and ritualistic practice, organizational and professional culture, management style, and technology and fluctuations in demand. All these may exert considerable influence over the extent to which an optimal skill mix can be achieved. Having determined the skills required, it is essential to consider their context in a group environment (group dynamics), since the bringing together of skills does not in itself ensure their effective functioning. The characteristics of the group must be such to ensure that the group is effective. An effective group is one that is likely to have developed a flexible structure, interactive relationships, strong and sensitive leadership and cohesive methods of operation that are relevant to the requirements of the work.

An optimum skill mix will be achieved when the desired standard of service is provided, at the minimum cost, consistent with the efficient deployment of trained, qualified and supervisory personnel and the maximization of contributions from all staff members. It will ensure the best possible use of scarce professional skills to maximize the service to clients (Nessling 1990).

DETERMINING SKILL MIX

Determination of skills and the mix of skills to meet patients' needs cannot be separated from individual, group, organization, economic and environmental factors. The NHS, with its numerous reorganizations, has introduced new structures, roles, and objectives and in doing so has paid little attention to some important factors affecting skill mix such as motivation, satisfaction, role clarity, job design and human resource management. Increased productivity, with goals for efficiency and effectiveness, form the main philosophy of the NHS reforms, as managers (clinician and general) strive to deliver this, serious thought must also be given to the human consequences of this new and, some believe, aggressive philosophy. Cooke postulates that the driving force and control necessary for achieving both high productivity and creative, flexible and adaptive behaviour is stored within the individual, who has made an emotional investment in some or all aspects of the organization's goals and methods (Cooke 1991). A practical example of this would be that the implementation of skill mix changes may demonstrate short-term benefits to the organization through the efficient management of the clinical resource. In the longer term, staff dissatisfaction and low motivation may have a detrimental effect on those benefits, if restructuring fails to consider that performance can be affected by the informal and formal relationships that exist between members of the health care team. Mumford makes clear the relationship between job satisfaction and skills use when she noted that job satisfaction is the fit between how an individual's skills are being used by an organization and how he wants these skills to be used (Mumford 1972).

Traditional manpower planning considered workers very much as a mass. Recent trends have changed the emphasis to integrate, in so far as is possible, the individual's and the organization's needs to ensure work motivation and satisfaction. This process is called 'human resource management'. Human resource planning is a crucial part of that process.

There are a number of stages to address when beginning to plan a skill mix for a particular service:

1 The existing situation must be established to determine if the current organization and staffing effectiveness can be improved. This

information should also incorporate job analysis, grading review (whether the right skills are applied to the relevant grade) and current performance, using performance management and appraisal. An analysis of existing staffing resources is essential (skills audit), where detailed personnel information would provide the basis for analysis of the strengths and weaknesses of the current workforce. It is also important to estimate any likely changes in resources, for example, loss of staff, supernumerary status of students, difficulties in recruitment due to demographic effect, staff returning from development courses etc.

2 Forecasting the skill requirements necessary to achieve service needs and targets is a difficult but necessary task. The use of staff activity analysis information, retrospective and prospective workload measurement, auditing of use of present skills and expertise and the effectiveness of their application will all provide useful information to make forecasting decisions.

3 A series of measures are necessary to ensure that effective deployment takes place at a local level, to ensure that the required skilled resources are available as and when required. This can be controlled by supply and demand variance (roster and workload monitoring), sickness and absence monitoring, holiday controls etc. Planning will assist the service to foresee changes and identify trends in staff resources, enabling the organization to respond quickly and to adopt policies that avoid difficulties for operational management, for example, identifying minimum safety levels and identifying skills that must be available at all times to provide a safe, quality service. Both strategic and operational planning must provide the clinical manager with the ability to reconcile differences between supply and demand at all times.

Planning the clinical resource provides clinicians with the opportunity to:

☐ assess the demands being placed on the service

☐ redefine roles and responsibilities

☐ reprofile the workforce

☐ reallocate resources to areas of greatest need

☐ review the effectiveness, efficiency and appropriateness of service provision.

METHODOLOGIES USED TO DETERMINE SKILL MIX

Traditionally studies focusing on manpower planning have made considerable efforts to determine the number of staff required, but seldom have the skills, or mix of skills, required to provide good quality care for patients been studied. There is no universally accepted methodology to determine skill mix. Many attempts are made to quantify and qualify the skills necessary to meet a given or anticipated demand. Techniques available are limited, and are themselves open to question as to the accuracy and validity of the information they provide. The techniques for the assessment of skill use, in an attempt to determine what skills are necessary, form two types of method. A 'top-down' approach using professional judgement or statistical analysis using manpower data, activity (bed occupancy) and cost have been commonly used to determine the number of staff needed. These methods are simple and cheap to apply. The disadvantages, however, are that the methodology assumes that bed occupancy equates to patient demand, regardless of patient care needs, and the skills required to undertake the work is not considered. As the top-down approach focused largely on the service in the macro sense, pressures from health care professionals increased to introduce 'bottom-up' objective measurement to reflect more readily local requirements so as to encourage ownership of information at the grass roots level where it was to be collected, and thus stimulate its management to improve resource uses. The introduction of work study analysis under the more professionally acceptable guise of 'staff activity analysis' and demand methodologies are increasingly being introduced. When carried out correctly, staff activity studies have certainly been helpful in identifying areas of skills wastage, but it must be remembered that lessons learnt from the use of work study demonstrate that task analysis in isolation does not succeed in solving the problems of managing the worker and work. What work study fails to capture is often as important as what it does capture. It does not analyse human behaviour, group interaction, managerial behaviour or the work environment; all key elements in understanding work, productivity, and the individual.

STAFF ACTIVITY ANALYSIS

Staff activity analysis uses two approaches, the first observes staff activity, with data collection carried out by trained observers, and second, self recording activity analysis, where the practitioners record their own activity. Both these methodologies record the activity of individuals in a specific time frame and this data can then be used to form the basis of analysis for skill mix determination. It is important to note at this point, that once staff activity and workload information (determined by using staff activity information combined in some cases with professional judgement to measure patient demand) is available, decisions to develop a skill mix to match demand will, in the main, be a professional and managerial one, and thus of a subjective nature. There remain differing views as to the relative importance of objective and subjective information. The Operational Research Service has documented a number of methods for determining demand measurement (ORS 1983). The report suggested that the best methods may well be those which have both a scientific base and incorporate professional judgement. Telford, who pioneered work on subjective methodologies for skill mix determination, said of the more objective methods that there may be an initial impression that solution to the nursing problem can be produced merely by calculation, and that the 'objective' methods were seen as more appropriate, but it does not take long however to realize that in each 'objective' methodology professional judgements are exercised at some stage or other in the assessment process.

In nursing, much energy has been placed on determining skill mix through activity analysis of one form or other, while acting on this information to achieve benefits has been rather more difficult. a discrete methodology-centred attempt to determine skill mix has probably imposed limitations on its potential development thus far. In conjunction with staff activity analysis, much work now needs to be carried out with all professional groups to determine job analysis and design, and to ensure role clarity, particularly in the aftermath of grading reviews and devolved management structures.

The challenge that skill mix poses for clinical managers is to integrate the needs of the organization, the needs of the patient, and the needs of the practitioner.

JOB ANALYSIS AND DESIGN

Job analysis and design has a number of aims, the primary aim being to satisfy the requirements of the organization for productivity, operational efficiency and quality of service. In addition, it aims to satisfy the needs of the individual, to provide challenge and the optimum use of skills and self-fulfilment. The process of job design must come from an analysis of the work to be done and the tasks or processes that need to be carried out for the organization or organizational unit to achieve its objectives. This is where the techniques of work study become useful. It is important to establish a robust job design from work requirements rather than designing a job purely for professional or managerial advantage, however, jobs must be designed and re-designed to facilitate challenge and the full use of the individual's skills, so in that sense a job may well be developed for an individual with special skills. A further aim of job design should be to address the needs of the individual performing the job. Katz argues that job satisfaction is a pathway to high productivity and to high quality production, and that the job itself must provide sufficient variety, sufficient complexity, sufficient challenge and sufficient skill to engage the abilities of the worker (Katz 1964).

Whilst information on staff activity and workload can be used as a broad indicator to determine how clinical time and skill is and should be utilized, skill mix analyses tend to maintain a fairly traditional view of the tasks to be undertaken by the different grades of staff in determining how many staff are required at each level, and focusing on local care delivery rather than total service delivery. Reprofiling can take this process one stage further and looks at whether, with additional training, certain tasks could be performed by some other grade or type of staff, and relates the service provided to the demand for that service by the consumer.

The issues surrounding skill mix will continue to be highly contentious, and the various interest groups will seek to either welcome or reject attempts (depending on the benefits or otherwise) to examine the different combinations of staff to determine an effective skill mix. To work towards the achievement of optimal skill mix professionals will need to ensure:

☐ that a reappraisal of present working practices takes place;

☐ accurate and valid information is available on resource use to support decision-making;

☐ further development of multi-professional collaboration to minimize the duplication of activity and skills wastage;

☐ the development of a more flexible workforce to enable maximum benefit from resource allocation to be realized;

☐ a reduction in professional protectiveness and self interest when at 'odds' with organizational objectives to improve patient care.

Skill mix determination cannot be carried out in a vacuum; the organization must play its part and will need to ensure:

☐ clear vision and objectives are communicated to all;

☐ realistic job design takes place;

☐ role clarity;

☐ purposeful selection for job;

☐ adequate training and development;

☐ individual job satisfaction;

☐ performance management with acceptable reward strategies;

☐ wide consultation with staff.

Reprofiling

Reprofiling describes the process used to develop new and more creative and innovative staffing structures with skill mix determination being a central part of that process. Reprofiling, as the name suggests, studies the current 'profile' of a part or whole service, and makes recommendations for its restructuring if necessary. The aim of reprofiling is to achieve the maximum use of skills and qualifications of each member of staff, within a framework that encompasses all activity, placing greater emphasis on the total service being provided with the patient as the focal point. Reprofiling, therefore, examines current structures, roles and responsibilities in the light of the need/demand for the service. The current trend towards a market-oriented approach to the provision of health care has led to increasing pressures to demonstrate that the highest possible quality service is being provided within available resources. The decision to reprofile a team or service will be determined by a number of factors:

☐   changing demand for the service or skills

☐   changing roles of clinical team

☐   changing supply of skills

☐   pressures for increased flexibility from staff and consumers

☐   introduction of support posts to professionals

The intention of undertaking a reprofiling exercise is to develop a structure that enables the most effective possible use of staff in providing the quality and level of service required to meet current and future needs within available resources. It supports the establishment of staffing structures that will allow staff to develop their roles. Reprofiling aims to increase the job satisfaction of staff by ensuring that these roles make full use of their level of skill, abilities and qualifications. A process of review is necessary to ensure that the correct balance of staff is maintained and that management and professional practices remain responsive to ongoing changes. Reprofiling must provide the opportunity for role enhancement and an improvement in the quality of service delivery.

Both skill mix and reprofiling have become critical resource management issues, as resources and deliverable targets become paramount in a value for money, cost constrained environment. Since a changing work environment has human as well as resource implications, the human aspects of implementing change must be considered carefully. Effective management of the change process is crucial for the implementation of lasting change. Approaches and techniques that can be used will be considered in Chapter 5.

Collaborative work within and between health care services is of the utmost importance to ensure effective, continuous health care delivery. Each discipline, therefore, cannot be viewed in isolation and the skills of the whole health care team (professional and support staff) need to be reviewed to take account of changing roles and responsibilities; as well as changing health care needs and demands.

CONCLUSION

Much of managing the human resource is about managing people at work, understanding their needs, supporting them in using the skills they have, and maximizing their potential. An effective manager sees each member of staff as an individual, and makes every effort to understand what it is they enjoy and dislike about their work, what flexibility they need or want and what their personal and professional aspirations are. To ensure that an adequate supply of staff is available it is necessary first, to determine the demand for the clinical workforce and second, to ensure that the demand is met by an adequate supply of resources.

ACTION GUIDELINES

The following guidelines will help you identify the significant areas for action in your clinical service:

1 Review your organization's manpower strategy

☐ how does it address your local supply needs?

☐ identify information requirements to determine local needs in relation to demand.

2 Conduct a skills audit

☐ establish current skills

☐ discuss with staff: - what they enjoy about their work
- what they dislike about their work
- their development needs

3 Review strengths and weaknesses of the current skills supply with your team

4 Identify mechanisms to minimize weaknesses and build on strengths

REFERENCES

Cooke P (1991) Human resource management, management briefing *Sheffield Business School* 17, October.

Drucker P (1989) *The Practice of Management.* London: Pan Business Management.

Katz D (1964) The motivational basis of organisational behaviour *Behavioural Sciences* **9**: 131.

Mumford E (1972) *Job Satisfaction: A Study of Computer Specialists*. London: Longman.

Nessling R (1990) *Manpower Monograph No. 2, Skill Mix: A Practical Approach for Health Professionals*. London: DoH/MPAG.

ORS (Operational Research Service) (1983) *Nurse Manpower Planning: Approaches and Techniques*. London: DHSS.

FURTHER READING

☐ Regional Consortium (Five Regions) (1991) *Using Information in Managing the Nursing Resource, A Learning Programme*. Macclesfield, Cheshire: Greenhalgh & Co. Ltd. Modules of particular relevance are: Skill Mix Management and Human Resource Management.

☐ Pearson R (1991) *The Human Resource: Managing People and Work in the 1990s*. London: McGraw-Hill.

☐ Walsh M and Ford P (1989) Nursing Rituals: *Research and Rational Actions*. Oxford: Heinemann.

ORGANIZATIONAL CHANGE & SERVICE DEVELOPMENT 5

Like everything else, organizations change over time. Some change rapidly, some change slowly. Some change in ways that make them more effective and some change in ways which make them less so. As the NHS develops to meet the needs of future health care provision, those involved in changing roles within a changing environment must recognize that change takes time especially where new attitude formation and new values are involved. Change can be threatening and support must be provided for those staff who may find initial difficulty in coping with new initiatives and more complex roles.

CHAPTER AIMS

☐ To present organization development and change issues in a way which sets them into the framework of the current climate within the NHS

☐ To identify typical reasons for change, and resistance to change

☐ To examine the theoretical and practical approaches that may be used to inform the change process

CONTEXT

Organizational change may happen in a variety of dimensions. The most immediately obvious are structural changes – reorganizations. However, changes may also occur in organizational processes, procedures, the people who fill key positions, technology, size and so on. Some changes can have a strong 'demand character' – that is, they are responses to other changes, either within or outside the organization which can hardly be avoided. Technological changes, for instance, may force the creation of new specialist roles and the granting of authority to those who fill them, or new computers requiring new expertise for their use. In contrast to these 'demand character' changes, many changes are made not because they are required, but because they seem desirable. They occur at somebody's discretion. Changes are typically initiated by key managers; they are top-down changes. There are also a number of change procedures grouped primarily under the title of 'organization development', that are more bottom-up, or at least the source of change is very close to where the change is applied.

Organization development is concerned with the diagnosis of organization health and performance, and with the implementation of programmes of planned change. It is a generic term embracing a wide range of intervention strategies into the social processes of the organization. These intervention strategies are aimed at the development of individuals, groups and the organization as a total system. Organization development is based on applied behavioural science. It concerns itself among other things with attitude formation and change, interpersonal skills and sensitivity training and with such methods and techniques as motivational processes, patterns of communication, styles of leadership, job enrichment and managerial behaviour.

Our present society is changing rapidly. The changes have a direct impact on the National Health Service. The advances in technology, markets, economic and environmental considerations, employee and customer expectations, demands for the service to be more user responsive, are just some of the forces on the service which make change even more dynamic. Organization development aims to address the difficulties involved in dealing with rapid and indeed discontinuous change. It is the term used to describe efforts designed and planned to improve the organization's overall effectiveness and not just improvements to a part or parts of the organization in isolation. Organization development efforts involve transforming the organization from one which resists change to one which deliberately promotes and plans needed change in order to adapt itself to new situations. In this way it helps the organization's ability to cope with, and adapt to, change. It is not limited to large organizations, but has as much relevance to small ones.

The focus of organization change

The National Health Service, like business and other care organizations is made up of a number of interrelated, interdependent parts, e.g. administration, clinical services, estates and facilities. The problems of integration and communication are of prime concern. The new focus is essentially upon how the service actually operates and how this is reflected in:

☐ the communications within the provider unit and with its external environment;

☐ the integration of the parts of the service and their interrelationships, ranging from the relation of the individual to his job, to the unit and its external environment (customers and consumers);

☐ the style of managing and the number of levels of supervision in the hierarchical structure.

Any organizational and service development effort should be designed to help the organization increase its effectiveness by improving its capacity to develop and use the capabilities of its people. To this end, people must be trained to function both as individuals and as members of working groups in how tasks are completed, i.e. on the process as well as the outcome, so that examination of the decision-making, planning, and communication processes becomes a normal way of working. It is for these reasons that the emphasis is placed on people and the need to increase their contribution, commitment and satisfaction within the organization. The purpose then of service development initiatives will be to:

☐ create a climate in the organization where it is better able to deal with its present and future problems;

☐ increase the organization's capacity to change when it needs to;

☐ make more effective use of people by helping them improve their ways of working;

☐ improve collaboration between different parts of the organization for more effective achievement of common objectives;

☐ create conditions whereby appropriate information can be channelled to those parts of the organization where effective decisions can be made;

☐ help create opportunities in which employees can make an effective contribution to organizational goals.

Approaching change and service development

It would be wrong to convey the impression that organization development and change involves a simple set of techniques which can easily and quickly be applied to solve day-to-day business problems. Rather it is a process which goes through several stages – diagnosis, planning necessary changes, implementation and review – all of which takes time. The diagnostic stage for example, involves an examination of the present organization and its ways of working, in the context of its present and future corporate objectives. Among the methods which can be used are individual interviews, group interviews and self-completion questionnaires. From this stage, a number of potential areas for change are identified and the implications are examined so that members of the organization can plan how to bring about the necessary changes. A strategy for change should also be evolved by the most senior managers, which enables implementation of change with the necessary control and review. Sometimes at the beginning of a change programme, given the need for qualified and competent resources to advise on change processes, external management consultants may be commissioned. At this time, outside advice could be invaluable for two specific reasons. First, it could offer skills and advice not available within the organization, and second, it could help develop internal resources to avoid over-dependence on external help. The main tasks involved would be to plan what action should be taken in the organization, so that the change process can get under way. Such actions should identify the changes necessary and help the organization assess and implement its own solutions. The impetus for change and development effort is provided by certain needs which arise within the organization, for example, the need:

☐ for adaptation to a new environment;

☐ to change structures and roles;

☐ to improve inter-group collaboration;

☐ for coping with problems of a merger or amalgamation;

☐ to open up communication systems;

☐ for better planning;

☐ to change 'cultural norms', since managing culture will be based on certain values, ground rules, norms, and power structure;

☐ to make the organization climate more consistent with both individual needs and the changing needs of the environment.

Change and organization development in the NHS

The NHS is not alone in having to grapple with the challenge of discontinuous and rapid change. Admittedly it is unique because of its sheer size and complexity. However, small and large scale organizations in the private sector are having to face similar challenges in terms of securing their future viability. Managers in a rapidly changing environment are having to develop good strategic vision. Keleher and Cole (1989) argue the need for this strategic approach in identifying the key issues in the external and the internal environment.

EXTERNAL NHS ENVIRONMENT: STRATEGIC ISSUES

Social changes

Examples are:

☐ rapidly rising numbers and proportions of elderly

☐ social mobility

☐ rise of the nuclear family

☐ more women working

☐ reduction in natural family/community support

☐ effects of long term unemployment

☐ north—south divide

☐ future changes in labour market

☐ lifestyle associated (alcohol, diet, smoking)

☐ AIDS

Technology

Examples are:

☐ increasingly sophisticated and expensive clinical equipment (scanners, monitors, life support)

☐ need for skilled staff to operate, interpret results from and maintain new clinical hardware

☐ advances in information technology

☐ complex laboratory analyses

☐ new pharmaceuticals

☐ new therapies

☐ advances in new rehabilitation techniques

Economics

Examples are:

☐ uncertainty in financial allocations

☐ opportunities (and threats) of new developments in funding the service

☐ macro-economic trends

Politics

Examples are:

☐ initiatives such as 'community care'

☐ changing priorities for initiatives, e.g. attention shifting from acute to community care

☐ introduction of competitive tendering

☐ impact of government plans on managing the NHS

☐ short-termism

☐ development of alternative providers of traditionally NHS care

INTERNAL NHS ENVIRONMENT: STRATEGIC ISSUES

Resources/inputs

Examples are:

☐ financial squeeze puts pressure on level of service

☐ problems in retention of staff

☐ professional 'de-tribalism'

☐ future of professions

☐ wider range of professions

☐ skill level and mix

Activity/process

Examples are:

☐ move away from 'repair of casualties' towards 'health promotion and maintenance'

☐ need for 'person-centred' team approach across professions

☐ influence of general management and NHS review

☐ incorporation of non-medical views in service planning

Performance/outputs

Examples are:

☐ lack of meaningful measures of outcome

☐ rise in consumerism

☐ role of media in influencing internal perceptions of the NHS

☐ inadequate 'information systems' imposed from the centre

Against the backdrop of the conceptual thinking behind the need for change and the empirical evidence provided by the behavioural scientists, it would appear that there is a need to accept the proposition that growth and change are normal elements of the world. Events are constantly happening that are difficult to understand or indeed, that could have been predicted. This new reality affects thinking not only in business, but in life. Turrill suggests that perhaps there was once a time when it was possible to approach the future in an orderly fashion, to make quantifiable predictions, bring to bear rational argument, make judgements, allocate resources and to set and achieve targets without finding that plans were overturned before they had been put into action (Turrill 1989). He argues 'the external pressures on all organizations are severe and the pace of change shows no sign of slackening'.

Given constant reminding that change will continue to be rapid and discontinuous it seems that the issue for managers is twofold. First, an understanding of the change process is essential; and second, learning to manage the tension in a world where simple choices are not presented most of the time, means learning to manage conflicting alternatives and paradox.

The change process

The organization provides the framework within which change takes place. In the past the change process has been perceived in terms of discrete packages or projects associated with perhaps the opening of a new unit, the retraction of a service, the introduction of new structure or the development of a new set of procedures as a few common examples. There is now so much change which many perceive as being imposed, that change for most has become a way of life. Factors such as uncertain economic conditions, competition, political intervention, scarcity of natural resources and rapid development in information technology create an increasingly volatile environment. In order to ensure its survival and future success, the organization must be responsive to change, but what is more important is how change is managed.

The planned process of change in an organization is achieved through the use of behavioural science technology and theory. There are many models which underpin and provide a guiding frame of reference for any change effort. However, whilst they are not mutually exclusive, they all stem from the original thinking of Kurt Lewin (1958). According to Lewin, the first step in the process of change is *unfreezing* the present level of behaviour. Since the introduction of resource management, health care professionals are now needing to practise in an 'information culture'. Unfreezing in this context means raising awareness of the use of credible and timely information upon which to base decisions. It entails the examination of ritualistic practice and the appraisal of how clinical care is managed, including dependency studies, workload and rostering systems. The unfreezing might include a series of training sessions in which an objective for change was agreed from a more participative viewpoint. It would also include the data feedback from any activity analysis survey undertaken.

The second step, *movement*, is to take action that will change the social system from its original level of behaviour or operation to a new level. In a ward, this action could include developing a primary nursing approach to care, altering the skill mix and introducing flexible rostering, to name only a few general examples.

Refreezing, the third step, involves establishing a process that will make a new level of behaviour 'relatively secure against change'. The refreezing process may include different conforming patterns, such as collaboration rather than competition. To give an example, anecdotal evidence well illustrates the demarcation line that in the past existed between day and night staff. To bring about lasting change in this sphere would mean, according to Lewin, initially unlocking or unfreez-ing the present social system. This requires a process of re-education. Behavioural movement must occur in the direction of desired change, such as the ward manager having 24-hour managerial responsibility for the ward and the introduction of internal rotation of staff. Finally, deliberate steps must be taken to ensure that the new state of behav-iour remains relatively permanent. Lewin's three-step approach is sim-ple to state. The implementation of this model is rather more difficult. Despite the difficulties, today's NHS presents many challenges and opportunities to learn in a new way, although traditional methods of learning will still be appropriate at times. In addition, managers are required to coach and be a mentor to their staff and to invest in learning technology. There may also be emotional issues to address such as stress, morale, suspicion, power, the need for open commu-nication and (not to be forgotten) the history of previous experiences of change.

Turrill describes a logical approach to change (1990). This is depicted in Table 5.1 below.

Table 5.1: Logical approach to change

Strategy	1 devise an overall strategy
Plan	2 turn the strategy into a plan
Implementation	3 seek sanction from those in authority
Changed behaviour	4 implement the plan

From Turrill (1990).

This process wrongly assumes that man is entirely a rational creature, who will therefore accept a well-reasoned, well-presented argument: if he resists, opposition can be overcome by the use of authority. Again wrongly, the assumption might be made that the existing organization has the competence and the capacity to work up the new arrange-ments.

Resistance to change

Changes do not always go according to plan. Indeed, some planned changes do not go through at all. Changes can meet resistance of a kind that stops them completely or, more frequently, diverts them in a direction other than anticipated. Some theorists imply that resistance to proposed change is irrational, that it arises from personality structures that are rigid, biased, authoritarian, and insecure. This can be true, but there are many instances when it is not.

Some proposed changes are poor ideas and not in the best interests of the organization. In such cases, rationality is on the side of the resistors. Change for its own sake has no inherent value; only change that contributes to the organization's goals is organizationally rational.

When resistance to change is referred to, the inference always seems to be that management is always rational and that employees are emotional or irrational in not responding in the way they should. If an individual feels he is going to be worse off as a result, any resistance is entirely rational in terms of his own best interest. In times of change, the interests of the organization and the individual do not always coincide. If not properly managed, change can decrease morale, motivation and commitment and create conflict within the organization.

There are individual characteristics inherent in those people who resist and those who embrace change. Table 5.2 below offers a comparison in a model adapted from Pym (1966).

In any planned change process, resistance will be less if:

☐ those affected by the change feel that the project is their own, not one imposed on them by outsiders;

☐ the change has the wholehearted support of top managers;

☐ the change is seen as reducing rather than increasing present burdens;

☐ the change accords with established values;

☐ the programme for change offers the kind of new experience which interests participants;

☐ participants feel that their autonomy and security are not threatened;

☐ participants have jointly diagnosed the problem;

☐ the change has been agreed by group decisions;

☐ those advocating the change understand the feelings and fears of those affected and take steps to relieve them;

☐ it is recognized that new ideas are likely to be misunderstood and ample provision is made for discussion of proposals to ensure complete understanding of them.

Table 5.2: Individual characteristics of change resisters and change embracers

Change resisters	Change embracers
Concern for safety and security	Desire for new experiences and some risk
Preoccupied primarily with means rather than ends	Greater attention to ends, less focus on means *per se*
Belief in 'a one best way'	Open to alternative courses of action
Aspire to regularity, order, financial security, prestige	Aspire to achievement, interesting work, freedom, personal responsibility
View managers as experts on work of their subordinates	View managers as generalists, not experts in all areas they supervise
Submissive with superiors and directive with subordinates	Emphasize authority appropriate to individual's contribution
Assume that old solutions once successful can be applied to new problems as well	Less stress on prior solutions and more concern with evidence related to specific problem at hand

Adapted from Pym (1966).

The changing role of clinicians in management

The development of the NHS reforms and the introduction of greater competition has brought about major changes to the traditional role of all NHS managers. This has had implications for the development of clinicians for future managerial responsibilities. In addressing the issues involved, the concept of culture is highlighted as a useful device for looking closer at the kinds of changes and channelled effort required towards achievement. Management is often described in terms of functions, such as planning, organizing, controlling and motivating. Mintzberg (1973) argues that in practice, however, managers perform up to ten roles, most of which involve short term horizons and fragmented activities. He further suggests that the mixture of roles differs from one managerial job to another, with factors such as organizational size and level in the hierarchy being important influences.

Close examination of the clinical manager's role as created in the first reorganization of the NHS in 1974 supports Mintzberg's views on the nature and variability of the managerial role. The role described in 1974 has changed and will continue to undergo further change in the future. Effective resource management reinforces the principle of general management at unit level. In many provider units the development of the resource management projects revolves around the creation of clinical directorates in all specialties. This has involved a complete change in organization structure to accommodate resource management. Even in units where directorate structures have not been implemented, the Trust status of providers opens the door on business planning, financial and activity targets and total quality management (TQM). The clinical manager's role of the future will require creative and innovative skills and managerial productivity which are congruent with a general management function. The emphasis is probably well placed on innovation.

Burns and Stalker's classic study of the management of innovation (1961) is a useful model. As provider units come to operate in a more competitive environment, clinical managers may experience some of the problems of adaptation as described by these writers. In Table 5.3 some probable changes are summarized. Although this is an oversimplification, as it is not suggested that all aspects of the old system should be discarded, it does highlight some important shifts of emphasis.

Table 5.3: Changes in systems of management

Aspects of management in provider units	'Old' systems	'New' systems (appropriate for dynamic competitive environment)
Objectives	Social	Commercial
Key tasks	Administration	Business planning
Promotion and power	Seniority, general skills and experience	Expertise, specialization and training
Structure	Centralized and bureaucratic	Decentralized and flexible
Planning	Short-term based on tradition	Long-term based on research
Decision-making	Rules and regulations	Greater personal initiative
Relationships	Status and individual roles	Job content and teamwork
Appraisal systems	Based on effective loyalty and criticism	Based on performance results and praise
Staff attitudes	Loyal and proud of the unit/hospital	Hopefully the same
Employment	Secure, well-paid, successful and caring	Striving for achievement to ensure success while still caring

In terms of organization change and development, and with reference again to the concept of culture, writers on organizations have compared one organization with another in efforts to define the attributes of success or lack of it. The envied success of Japanese industrial culture has further enhanced interest in the culture concept. Edgar Schein (1980) describes culture as 'the pattern of basic assumptions which a given group has invented, discovered or developed in learning to cope with its problems of external adaptation and internal integration, which have worked well enough to be considered valid and, therefore, to be taught to new members as the correct way to perceive, think and feel in relation to those problems'. This almost has a scientific ring to it! From another angle, Charles Handy (1979) examines culture managerially and perceives a presence within organizations of particular managerial philosophies, styles or cults. In this context, organizations develop their own cultures, always some mixture of the basic cult, since few organizations are culturally pure. Handy's theory of cultural propriety describes using a blend as a way of mixed rather than mixed up management. Whilst the concept of culture is a popular one in the literature, it does not provide a panacea for management. It must be viewed as a complex and multidimensional concept which can be a useful guide in establishing organization development needs. As the NHS develops to meet the needs of future health care provision, those involved in changing and developing their role within a changing organization must recognize that change takes time and certainly will not happen overnight, especially when new attitude formation and new values are involved. This is a salient point as perhaps the dominant culture existing in parts of the NHS has encouraged people who are conservative in their attitude to change. Change can be threatening and support must be provided for those managers who may find initial difficulty in coping with a more complex role. A quote from Mikhail Gorbachev provides an apt and final comment for change agents:

Life style cannot be changed in the twinkling of an eye, and it is harder still to put an end to inertia in thinking.

CONCLUSION

It is through the process of management that the efforts of members of the organization are co-ordinated and guided towards the achievement of organizational goals. Management is the cornerstone of organizational effectiveness. In addition to arrangements for carrying out organizational processes and the execution of work, management has the responsibility for creating an organizational climate in which people are motivated to work willingly and effectively. Organizational climate is a general concept and difficult to define precisely. It can be said to relate to the strength of feelings of belonging, care and goodwill among members of the organization. A healthy climate will not by itself guarantee organizational effectiveness, unless the climate evokes a spirit of co-operation and is conducive to motivating members to work willingly and effectively. There is a wide range of interrelated individual, group, organizational and environmental influences on behaviour, and therefore many different criteria which might be applied in an attempt to assess organization performance and effectiveness. An organization must also be properly prepared to face the demands of a changing environment. It must give attention to its future development and success. Any work organization can only perform effectively through interactions with the broader external environment of which it is part. Factors such as the level of government intervention, consumer responsiveness and rapid developments in new technology create an increasingly volatile environment. In order to ensure its future success and survival, the organization must be readily adaptable to the external demands placed upon it. The organization must be responsive to change. What is also important is how change is handled, that is, the management of change. This chapter has highlighted the complex issues in change management and the nature of the people–organization relationship. Chapter 6 is devoted to an approach to work organization that offers a structured way to managing assignments as part of the change process.

ACTION GUIDELINES

The following guidelines will help you to identify the significant areas for action in your clinical service:

I   List five 'changes' that you have had to introduce or help introduce at work. This could include changes in work methods, the introduction of new jobs or tasks, changes in responsibilities, procedures, etc.

2   For each 'change' try to sum up your own staff's initial attitude to the change

3   From the changes you list, take the one that was initially at least received with some level of resistance. Try to identify the 'factors' that you believe caused your staff to hold such attitudes. Be as honest as you can

4   Now take another change from your list, but this time take one that was received with some level of acceptance. Again, try to list the factors that you believe caused your staff to hold such attitudes

5   Having reflected on your experience of change, identify a maximum of three key points to which you believe managers should pay attention

6   You should now try to establish what these key points mean in relation to developing into a more effective manager. Try to identify:

☐   What additional knowledge and understanding you will need

☐   What new skills and abilities you will need to develop

☐   What changes in attitude will be needed by your staff

REFERENCES

Burns T and Stalker G M (1961) *The Management of Innovation*. London: Tavistock.

Handy C (1979) *Gods of Management*. London: Pan Books Ltd. 1979.

Keleher R and Cole E (1989) Strategy and the NHS – Do we need it? *Health Service Management* 73–76, April.

Lewin K (1958) *Group Decision and Social Changes: Readings in Social Psychology*. New York: Holt, Rhinehart and Winston.

Mintzberg H (1973) *The Nature of Managerial Work*. New York: Harper and Row.

Pym D (1966) Effective managerial performance in organizational changes *Journal of Managerial Studies*, February.

Schein E H (1980) *Organisation Psychology*. Englewood Cliffs, NJ: Prentice Hall.

Turrill A (1989) *Resource Management – Changing the Culture*. Occasional Papers. London: NHS Training Authority. February.

Turrill A (1990) *Change and Innovation. A Challenge for the NHS*. London: The Institute of Health Services Management.

FURTHER READING

☐ Handy C (1989) *The Age of Unreason*. London: Arrow Books Ltd.

☐ Lewin K (1958) *Group Decision and Social Change: Readings in Social Psychology*. New York: Holt Rhinehart and Winston.

☐ Mintzberg H (1973) *The Nature of Managerial Work*. New York: Harper and Row.

☐ Wright S (1989) *Changing Nursing Practice*. London: Edward Arnold.

A PROJECT MANAGEMENT APPROACH TO WORK

6

Project management is recognized as a specialist branch of management which has evolved in order to co-ordinate and control some of the complex activities of modern industry. It is not an isolated example of a management skill acquired through the necessity created by industrial development and expansion. One of the fundamental and most familiar aspects of everyday life is the growth of living things. This growth can be observed in a single plant, in a baby animal or more widely, in a whole colony or population. Competition for available food, water and shelter must intensify as more mouths or roots require feeding. The effects of climate and other predators add other elements of risk. In the course of time, only those organisms which are able to adapt themselves will manage to prosper. The rule of 'survival of the fittest' will reign, resulting in the evolution of life forms which grow more specialized as time proceeds.

☐ **To present the use of project management
approaches and techniques to everyday work**

☐ **To outline the project management
infrastructure, roles and responsibilities to
ensure effective management**

CONTEXT

The world of work organization suggests close parallels with the world
of nature when the effects of growth and evolution are compared.
Continuous development and adaption to change will create more
demand for all the available resources. Evolutionary processes must
occur to meet the challenges presented by their continually changing
environment and economic climate. Some organizations will emerge as
more successful than others, whilst those that cannot re-adapt will not
remain viable. The need for a project management approach to work is
now widely recognized in the NHS. This chapter offers ideas on how
managers can begin to develop project management skills. It is dedicated to the proposal that a good project manager can make a difference
and, the skills to become a good project manager can be learned.

A project is any complex task that involves numerous sub-tasks,
intricate scheduling and complicated monitoring techniques. It can
range from conducting a study, or introducing a new method of practice, to planning a conference or masterminding a corporate acquisition. Although many important jobs can be handled informally through
the master task, others require the kind of formal organization involved
in major initiatives like a new hospital build, or indeed the resource
management roll-out programme.

Projects in the context of everyday management

Everyday management is concerned with ensuring that a service is provided which continually meets agreed customer requirements within a given resource level, through the involvement of all those providing the service.

A service like the NHS is made up of a set of highly complex activities, which may represent a series of projects, some of which may be connected to each other, some may be discrete in their entity as special projects which are one-off. That said, no project should exist in isolation. Each should have a direct link to the organization's corporate mission. The objectives contained therein are translated into sub-objectives which then become individual managers' objectives, and performance related.

Project management: the structure

A project is an assignment or endeavour with a specific objective. It is most frequently a one-time effort. It has specific start and end dates and it is divisible into explicit phases. The management structure in projects is illustrated in Figure 6.1 and the roles of the people involved in the structure are discussed below.

THE PROJECT SPONSOR

All projects in the private and public sector organizations have sponsors. The sponsor provides the source of authority to the project manager. The project sponsor would normally be a senior manager. For large projects, the sponsor would be the unit general manager/chief executive. The sponsor is the source of leadership.

THE PROJECT STEERING GROUP

The role of the project steering group is to monitor the progress of the project. The group will meet on a regular basis as agreed in phase one of the project plan. The people involved in the steering group will represent all the services involved in the project and therefore will have the knowledge and the authority to contribute to its success. The steering group will be able to help resolve problems and bottlenecks.

THE PROJECT MANAGER

The project manager is a full or part-time role. The project manager is

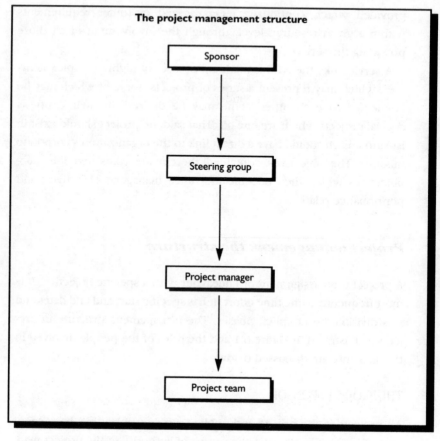

Figure 6.1: The project management structure

there to organize all those involved in the project, to meet its objectives and to anticipate and solve problems.

THE PROJECT TEAM

The team is responsible for carrying out the project as described in the project work plan. The team members might be in full-time roles for the duration of the project, or have part-time roles in the team on a co-opted basis.

Project management: a seven step approach

STEP ONE: SET THE GOAL

In this first stage the purpose of the project must be established. A concrete goal statement will underpin the project purpose. It is better to say 'the purpose of this project is to implement open visiting as a quality initiative' than 'the purpose of this project is to improve quality'. It is important also that the goal statement is clear, for two reasons. First, it identifies the overall purpose of the project as intended by the sponsoring manager and as understood by the project manager and second, this early clarification establishes in mutual agreement not only the task in hand, but also its ownership by the sponsor and delegation as a tasked objective to the project manager.

STEP TWO: SET A FINAL DEADLINE

At this early stage an end date should be set. If a final deadline has not been given then the project manager should set his own.

STEP THREE: IDENTIFY THE SUB-TASKS

It is important to break the project down into sub-tasks. This effort helps in defining the steps which are required to meet the goal of the total project exercise.

STEP FOUR: ORDER THE SUB-TASKS

The sub-tasks are organized into an appropriate order of performance. The start point is decided, then what comes next, then next and so on. Progression depends on both the nature of the sub-task and the appropriate time sequence. Some projects have a sequential line of development – meaning tasks are handled one at a time, with each one completed before the next one is started. Others have a parallel line of development – meaning several tasks are handled simultaneously.

STEP FIVE: SET TARGETS

Target dates and benchmarks are set. A deadline should be set for each sub-task. It is advisable to build in some extra time to cover delays or problems. It is often useful to set milestone points as well – specific review dates for evaluating overall progress and modifying the course of the project when necessary.

STEP SIX: ASSIGN SUB-TASKS

Sub-tasks are assigned to the **project manager** and to others involved. All possible sub-tasks should be delegated to project members and when feasible, specialists or other professionals on a co-opted basis. It is imperative that everyone knows his/her responsibilities and target dates. The project leader should add the tasks he/she will personally manage to the master list, transferring them to daily lists as appropriate.

STEP SEVEN: MONITOR PROGRESS

The monitoring process is on-going until the project is completed. It is useful to set up a project sheet, a list of all tasks, to whom delegated and due dates. These sheets can be kept in a folder for a daily check. The project leader should ensure his/her own jobs are being fed on to the daily list, following on with others as necessary. Completed tasks can be crossed off, thus visually highlighting any items that are lagging behind schedule.

Leadership in project management

A prototype role model for the project manager is illustrated in Figure 6.2.

In the informational role, the project manager acts as a monitor. Formal and informal channels of communication are exploited to gather intelligence about what is happening in the outside environment and within the team. As a disseminator of information, the project manager should ensure that there is good information for those who need it, both inside and outside the team. The project manager is also the spokesperson for the project team, the source of formal information to and on behalf of the group.

In the decisional role, the project manager is the one who decides

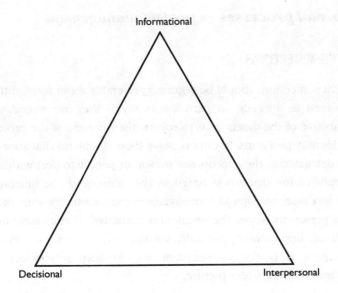

Figure 6.2: Prototype role model

on resource use and the allocation of tasks. Entrepreneurial skills encourage innovation, seek new opportunities and argue for new ideas with the sponsor and others as appropriate within the organization. The project manager also needs to be able to recognize and deal with conflict, and manage personal problems in the team should they arise. Negotiation is also a skill in this context as mutually beneficial work is agreed with staff.

At the interpersonal level, the project manager is a figurehead – the formal representation of the project at meetings, taking an 'official' role at the project team meetings. The role also involves liaison with peers and managers.

Finally, the project manager is responsible for the execution of the project. When planning is completed, the plan has to be put into effect. This can be a time of increasing pressure for the project manager. Successful execution is a combination of effective procedures and effective management. The right climate organizationally is an important support.

Formal processes in project management

REVIEW MEETINGS

Review meetings should be regular, (preferably about fortnightly), and planned in advance so participants know they are attending. The objective of the meetings is to review the progress of the project and to identify problems, but not to solve them. Problems that arise should be delegated to the appropriate person or people to deal with and the details of the delegation noted in the minutes of the meeting. The project manager should formally agree the measurable outcome with the person to whom the problem is delegated. Formal meetings provide an important opportunity for everyone to get an overview of progress. It is also an excellent way to keep sub-project leaders informed of the wider picture.

MILESTONES

Milestones are a vital indicator for the project manager. Early missed milestones must not be ignored. It is important to be clear about the answers wanted from people: '90% complete' is not accurate. 'How long to completion?' is the right question. If there are dependencies on outside support within the project, that progress should be reviewed regularly. Progress reports may be included in the project plan as a deliverable or contractual obligation.

COMPILING INFORMATION

Gathering relevant information is a combination of informal and formal processes. It includes asking for information about progress from the project team, maintaining contact with other departments, and following formal report procedures. Tracking and reporting progress involves communication with team members and managers if changes occur. Most importantly, the project sponsor needs to know how the project is progressing. The project team need to be informed individually and collectively. This is essential for their morale, to update their commitments and for feedback and evaluation if they as an individual have been delegated the responsibility for a sub-task.

CHANGING THE PROJECT

Change control is a central issue for the project manager. Controls should be in place before the execution stage of the project begins. The project manger must impose discipline in change matters, as uncontrolled changes are a major source of delay and failure in projects. Change control procedures involve deciding who will identify the need for changes, what format change requests should be made in, and who will approve changes. The following are suggestions of what would be subject to change control procedures:

☐ the project definition report

☐ the project milestones – both for the overall project and for the sub-projects

☐ the project plan

Changes to any of the above should be formally requested in writing using an established procedure. The project steering group will usually approve requests for change.

The project may be replanned within the change control mechanism, usually as a result of a change in project priority, a change in resources or a change in the project requirements. Replanning will be necessary if deliverables become significantly different or the project goal has been significantly amended from the original. A second reason for replanning is when the project is delayed so much that its links with other work is being affected. Yet a third reason is if morale is running low because of change or other problematic issues.

EVALUATION

When the project is complete, it is necessary to look at what worked and what did not. Evaluation of the project successes and failures at the end of the project is just as much an investment as the planning before it takes place. The project will be reviewed by the key players in the project – the team, other departmental representatives and managers as appropriate. The objective of evaluation is to learn from the experience, not to lay blame. It is therefore important to work through the evaluation process in the 'right climate'. This of course will be easier if the climate was right during the project.

Project management tools

THE PROBLEM-SOLVING PROCESS

The problem-solving process is a logical sequence for solving problems and improving the quality of decisions. The process can be applied to any problem or deviation from requirements, and can also be used to tackle an opportunity. Problems no matter their size or complexity can be solved through a sequence of steps. This ensures that everything possible will be done to apply the available resources in the most effective manner, to consider a number of options and to select the best solution.

In project management the problem-solving process can be used for:

☐ producing a clear statement of the identified problem or opportunity;

☐ gathering all necessary information associated with a problem or opportunity;

☐ analysing collected data and providing a clear statement of the root causes of the problem or the benefits of an opportunity;

☐ producing a list of all potential solutions to a problem or opportunity;

☐ selecting the best solution to fit the problem or opportunity;

☐ providing a plan for implementation;

☐ implementing and testing a plan;

☐ establishing a process for continuous improvement and holding the gains.

Two of the frequently used problem-solving techniques now follow as examples.

CREATIVE THINKING/MIND-MAPPING

This is a way of holding an individual brainstorm. The method makes deliberate use of word associations, encouraging the following of thought patterns wherever they may lead. It provides a written record of the output which can easily be summarized into a set of themes.

It can be used as an alternative to list-making for generating new ideas. It is particularly useful when it is felt that there are very few ideas or even none at all about a problem.

Method

1 Put the topic/issue/question at the centre of a clean sheet of paper. Draw a line around it.

2 Allow the mind to wander around the subject.

3 Starting with the first thought, draw a line from the centre and write down the second thought and similarly draw a line around it.

4 Do not pause. When one idea runs out, start a new one, with a new line out, to show the link.

5 Do not block the thoughts and do not evaluate. Put everything down that emerges in thinking about the central subject.

6 Do not worry about order or organization.

7 When all ideas are finally on the map, take a different colour pen and join up associated ideas.

Figure 6.3 shows a typical example of a mind map, illustrating the feasibility of flexible rostering.

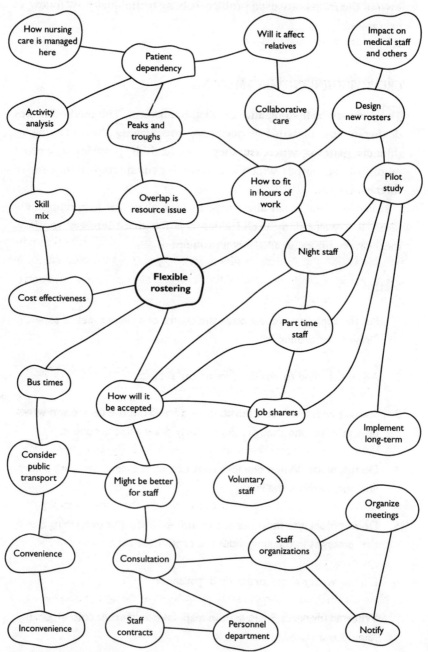

Figure 6.3: Mind map

The themes which are elicited from this particular brainstorm are:

- [ ] employee relations issues

- [ ] patient dependency issues

- [ ] cost effectiveness issues

- [ ] change management issues

SWOT analysis

This is a way of categorizing the related issues of a problem at status quo into the strengths, weaknesses, opportunities and threats that will be involved in solving the problem by change. Like the mind-map, it also provides a written record of the output which can then be summarized into a set of themes.

Method

1 Draw a vertical and a horizontal line to divide a clean sheet of paper into four areas and head each of the areas

   STRENGTHS   WEAKNESSES   OPPORTUNITIES   THREATS

2 Think through the problem and the potential changes that are needed to solve it.

3 List the issues related to the problem/change under each heading.

4 The exercise can require deeper thought either individually or collectively.

5 SWOT analysis is often used to formalize the thought process in problem solving after the problem has first been addressed in a mind map.

6 SWOT analysis has a credible place in formal written reports and documents.

Table 6.1 shows a typical example of a SWOT analysis: the implementation of a quality approach in the primary care setting.

Table 6.1: SWOT analysis: the project environment

Strengths	Weaknesses
Business management	Service contracting underdeveloped. Some unevenness
Computerized systems installed	
Beginnings of NHS marketing infrastructure	Some fragmented ill co-ordinated activities
Top management support	Underdevelopment of outcome and quality indicators
Well established links with other provider units	
	Some 'preciousness' with information by some actors
Project will complement the community	
	Discomfort with the strong axis of GP fundholding by some other provider agencies
Resource management project	
Highly motivated team within the practice	

Opportunities	Threats
Chance for a radical service review	'Project' approach is new
	Awareness of resource management is still being developed and understood
GPs can become more assertive and demanding of provider unit	
Stronger public health and intersectorial campaigns	The initiative is seen as extra work by clerical staff
Strengthen the doctor/manager interface	'Price of quality' concept not yet accepted/understood
Invasion of niche markets	Regional Health Authority involvement
Intelligent and critical learning of the resource management/quality interface	
	Gaps in practice may be exposed
Increase the focus on 'avoidance' of hospitalization	Resistance to change and development
A quality driven service	

WORK BREAKDOWN STRUCTURES

A work breakdown structure is the division of the entire job into logical groupings of related tasks. It is a graphic tool used to show how the project is structured. Each level should contain all the tasks of the job. Each level should be a logical expansion of the level above. Each should have a degree of detail and, should have a consistent organization (e.g. by discipline or product). Sub-division should continue down to the smallest logical task, i.e. the indivisible unit of work that can be assigned to an individual or a team.

A work breakdown structure essentially provides a structure for task identification in the project. It is the basis for bottom-up cost estimating. It is also the basis for network diagrams and it helps to avoid overlooking work segments and tasks. Figure 6.4 is an example of a work breakdown structure which might be used in a project which addresses the management of nursing care.

CRITICAL PATH SCHEDULING

Critical path scheduling is a network analysis technique which can be applied to the planning and control of project work. Within a project, there are operations which have the following common characteristics:

☐ Activities – the operations can be analysed into many separate activities, each taking time.

☐ Logic – the nature of the operation is such that some activities must precede others, and some are carried out in parallel.

☐ Resources – each activity requires some combination of resources – people, machines, material and money. Usually there is more than one possible combination of resources for any one activity.

The operations can be represented in a network diagram in which an arc represents an activity and a node represents an event (the start or finish of any one or more activities). The structure of the network illustrates the logical sequencing of the different activities. In order to create a network diagram, it is useful to compile what is known as a

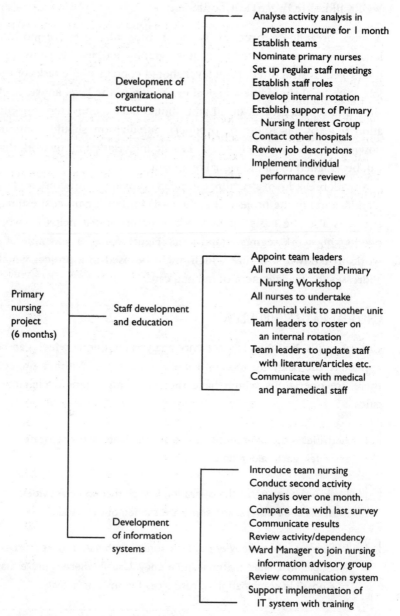

Figure 6.4: Work breakdown structure

precedence list. In this exercise, each of the tasks involved in the project is listed and identified by alphabetical letter and number. From this first list, those tasks which have to be carried out in order of priority because progress is dependent on their completion are again identified in list form. Subsequently, those tasks which can succeed the priorities are listed and finally, a timescale allocated to each task.

A critical path schedule provides details of the timing of activities and their requirements throughout the duration of the whole project. It directs attention to the critical activities which are not necessarily the larger jobs or the later jobs. During the project, progress information is used to update the schedule and produce a revised analysis.

Table 6.2 provides an example of a precedence list, Figure 6.5 is a network diagram used in a Nursing Dependency Study in a large acute hospital and Figure 6.6 is a representation of the project in Gantt chart form.

Table 6.2: Precedence List – Nursing Dependency Study

	Task		Predecessor	Successor	Duration (days)
Research	A	1	—	B C	15
Project goal	B	2	1 A	D E	1
Secure funds	C	3	1 A	O	40
Talk to managers	D	4	2 B	I F	20
Talk to staff	E	5	4 B	F	20
Define criteria	F	6	5 E	G H	20
Design spreadsheet	G	7	6 F	K	5
Recording forms	H	8	6 F	K	2
Link person profiles	I	9	5 D	J	1
ID link person	J	10	9 I	L	20
Modify criteria	K	11	6 H	L	20
Run pilot	L	12	11 K	P	20
Equipment	M	13	3 O	L	20
Accommodation	N	14	3 O	L	20
Team	O	15	3 C	M N	20
Draw up schedule	P	16	12 L	Q	5
Roll out	Q	17	16 P	—	—

GANTT CHARTS

The Gantt chart is a very simple, easy to use tool which illustrates in bars the period of time each task in the project should take. It is a

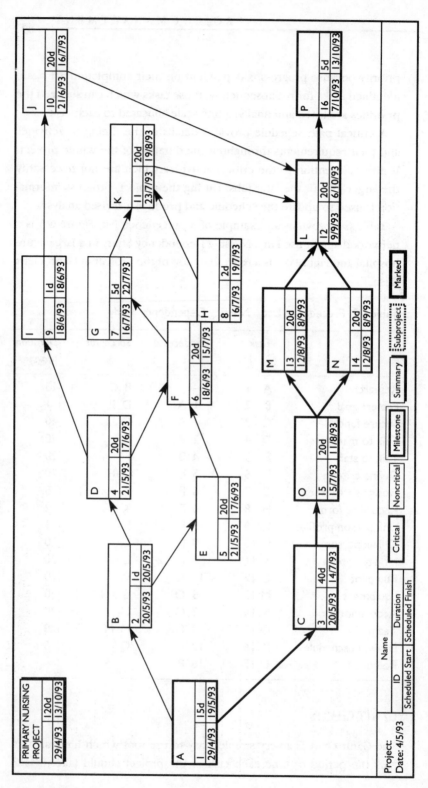

Figure 6.5: Critical path analysis

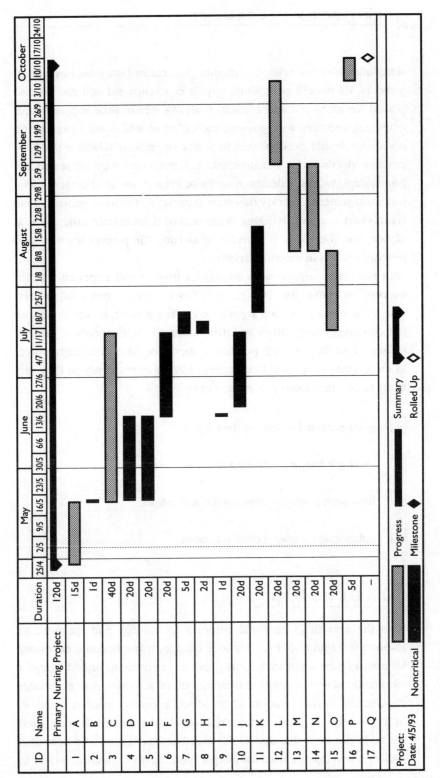

Figure 6.6: Gantt chart

ID	Name	Duration
	Primary Nursing Project	120d
1	A	15d
2	B	1d
3	C	40d
4	D	20d
5	E	20d
6	F	20d
7	G	5d
8	H	2d
9	I	1d
10	J	20d
11	K	20d
12	L	20d
13	M	20d
14	N	20d
15	O	20d
16	P	5d
17	Q	–

Project:
Date: 4/5/93

Progress   Summary

Milestone   Rolled Up

Noncritical

scheduling tool and is used to monitor and control the time element of projects. Its benefit is its simplicity. It is a visual aid and can be displayed for all to see and consult. It shows where time slippages are occurring and therefore gives an indication of when and where extra resources should be deployed to a task or, indeed whether the programme needs to be rescheduled. A Gantt chart may be scaled by hours, days, weeks, calendar months or even years. In short-term project management a weekly timescale is probably the most realistic. The Gantt chart is a 'live' working document to demonstrate progress at a glance, and therefore, is a means of alerting the project team to any potential delays in meeting targets.

In summary, anyone who manages a project will experience both success and difficulty. This chapter has covered a range of project management topics which are relevant to any project. It is by intention not comprehensive, rather an introduction to the elements of project management that through personal experience have been highlighted as important. They have been covered in an order in which they are likely to be encountered as projects proceed:

☐ getting started – defining the project

☐ making it happen – planning and organizing

☐ how we do things – organization and culture

☐ influencing people – communications

CONCLUSION

With the growth in new and complex technology and the need to respond to rapid and discontinuous change, it has become necessary for managers to adapt traditional structures in order to provide greater integration of a wide range of their functional activities. A flexible form of structure is the creation of groupings based on project teams in order to attain a specific managerial task. When the task is completed the team can be disbanded or the members reassigned to a new one. Project teams may be used for people working on a common task or to co-ordinate work on a specific project, such as the development of a new service. Project teams have been used in many organization systems and programmes. A project team is more likely to be effective when it has a clear objective, a well defined task, a definite end result to be achieved, and the composition of the team is chosen with care.

ACTION GUIDELINES

The following guidelines will help you develop some of the project management techniques discussed in the chapter:

1   You should be familiar with your organization's mission statement and corporate objectives. Access this information and share it with your colleagues

2   Write three personal objectives which relate directly to a corporate objective of your organization

3   Discuss the merits of the personal objectives identified in guideline 2 above with your manager. Choose the most appropriate for a project

4   Identify the problem areas using one of the problem-solving techniques

5   Produce a clear definition of your proposed project

6   Develop a project plan for action

FURTHER READING

☐ Lock D (1970) *Project Management.* Aldershot: Gower Press Ltd.

☐ Makower M S and Williamson E (1985) *Teach Yourself Operational Research.* London: Hodder and Stoughton.

☐ NHSME (1991) *Managing Resource Management Projects. Practical Experience.* London: Resource Management Unit, DoH.

☐ Winston S (1989) *The Organised Executive.* London: Kogan Page.

A FOCUS ON QUALITY IN PROVIDING CARE 7

Better quality services do not happen by accident, improvement requires reform, innovation and tough decisions

(Major 1991)

Charles Handy in his recent best seller tells the parable of the frog (Handy 1990). If a frog is immersed in water and slowly heated, the frog will eventually be boiled to death. The amphibian is too comfortable with continuity – the slow rise in temperature – to realize that continuous change at some point becomes discontinuous, and demands a change in the frog's behaviour. Unfortunately, the frog does not learn. This analogy can be used to describe quality in service organizations. Some organizations operate from the belief that what has always been done will be what they will always do; seemingly, they believe they are impervious to changes in their environment. A typical response to a problem is to identify whether the cause was doing too much or too little about the problem. That things could be done in a different way does not occur to them. Other organizations, recognizing the need to change embark on change programmes, yet fail to realize that the obstruction is the very thing they are trying to change – their culture. This is in itself problematic, as it is often believed that change is taking place, but in fact they are blind to their predicament.

CHAPTER AIMS

☐ To address the meaning of quality, with reference to current thinking and activity in the NHS

☐ To focus on the management of quality in cost control

CONTEXT

What is known about the introduction of quality management in the NHS, is that it requires, if it is to be successful a total cultural change. Quality management is not a discrete system, nor an education programme, nor a set of activities which place extra demands on time. Wherever this is the attitudinal stance, there is evidence of the temperature rising around the proverbial oblivious frog.

The implications for quality management

Since quality has had a raised profile in most organizations over the last decade, the focus has been shifted from the *provider* of the goods or services to the *consumer* or *customer* of those goods or services. In the manufacturing or retail industries this seems appropriate terminology and indeed escapes remark. However, in the care service environment, some people feel uncomfortable referring to patients or clients as 'customers' or 'consumers'.

Notwithstanding, the debate is one of pedantics. In managing a service which offers care, as resource intensive and part of the public sector as is the NHS, the identification of exactly *who* is the customer is crucial for any manager involved in quality initiatives. In the past it has been easy to regard patients as the customers in their being the receivers of a particular package of care. In this sense they are what is termed the *external customer*. However, in the context of any area within the NHS where one agency is making a contribution to the whole complex process involved in the management of a hospital or a community unit, there are a whole host of people known in the quality management world as *internal customers*. All NHS staff if asked would say that the patients or clients are their customers, and ultimately they are. In the provision of any service there is a chain of events which has to occur in order to achieve an overall objective or goal. If the laundry service in a hospital is used as an example, Figure 7.1 illustrates the chain of events involved in that particular process.

Whilst this model is over-simplistic it illustrates the concept of the internal customer. The customers of the laundry staff are the users of

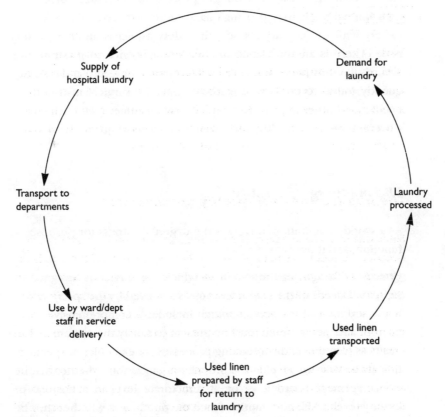

Figure 7.1: A system of supply

the linen at ward/department level, as are the porters who transport the supplies to the venue of order. The users of the linen similarly are customers of the portering staff. At the point of care delivery the patient becomes everyone's customer. In organizations committed to quality this perception of the internal customer is quite clear. Each agency involved in the process of care delivery appreciates and understands each other's role, with the main aim being to provide a quality service within resource. In hospitals, a common complaint of nurses is about the lack of items of linen. The laundry manager's problem in this context is often not that his staff are unable to process more linen to despatch to a ward (which might be the nurse's perception) rather, that the linen is unavailable due to its non-return of many items for whatever reason. This 'shrinkage' as it is known in stock control terms is the actual issue. In ensuring that linen is not stockpiled but returned and retained in the system for the process to continue, nurses can contribute directly to improving quality at no extra cost. Similarly, and to stay with the laundry service, the safety aspect is another quality issue. There is an abundance of anecdotal evidence to illustrate the hazards to safety because laundry is ill-prepared for return and is subsequently found to contain dangerous items like surgical instruments, needles and other objects. Healthy internal customer relationships are a prerequisite for a healthy organization in terms of quality service.

The meaning of quality

As a working definition, quality is the degree of fitness for purpose or function, and it has two aspects:

Quality of design, or the extent to which the service is designed to satisfy the needs of the customer. This is achieved by the *specification* – a description of the service which includes a comprehensive statement of all aspects which must be present to satisfy the customer. The business planning and contracting processes are examples of specification at the strategic level in the provider organization, whether that be at management board level or at directorate level in a hospital or locality level in the community. Since the purchasers whether they be District Health Authorities or GP Fundholders now contract with providers for services on behalf of patients, quality measures can be written into those contracts. A GP can place a contract with a hospital for a number of hip replacements and in so doing agree details like the time the patient will wait between referral and the first out-patient appointment. Cost of treatment and a protocol for receiving information on discharge are two further examples of specification that would be included in a contract.

Quality of conformance to design, or the extent to which the specification is actually achieved – the function of the processes which are used to produce the service. As yet this aspect of quality is not as well developed in the NHS as it is in many service organizations. It is however, a dimension of quality which has implications in the effective use of resources.

If one were to visit one of the well-known restaurant chains, it would be reasonably easy to recognize their set procedure when serving customers. The order is taken for beverages, and they are served. The order is taken for food and it is served. Part of the way through the meal a member of the waiting staff checks that the customer is satisfied with the meal. On receipt of the bill the customer pays and eventually leaves the restaurant having had a clear indication of how a complaint could be lodged if standards had not been achieved. In the NHS standard setting, customer satisfaction surveys and other quality initiatives being implemented address the improvement of the service. However, it is arguable that they are discrete activities better developed in some pockets of the service than others. When the activities are co-ordinated on an organization-wide basis, the real issue of achieving the specification is addressed, and *continuous quality improvement* will realize this.

There are certain caveats to be noted. Service quality is more difficult for the consumer to evaluate than goods quality. This is so for two reasons. First, service quality involves the subjective response of the consumer. It is not an absolute. Second, quality evaluations are not made solely on the outcome of a service. They also involve evaluations of the process of service delivery.

In order to manage service quality, it is necessary to know the consumer's view of it. This in turn requires the service provider to ascertain what criteria the consumer uses in evaluating service quality.

These are the quality determinants. Furthermore, the way in which the consumer's perception of quality arises is a key issue.

Total quality management

The Japanese were the first to discover that the most important job in a business is to continuously improve quality. They realized that quality is the key to success and understood that it depends on:

☐   the commitment of top management

☐   the efforts of all employees

As early as 1927 the Americans had begun to use statistical methods to improve their weapons, but met with failure because management commitment and understanding was lacking. Many firebombs dropped by the United States during the second world war failed to explode. They were found to be defective, and led the Japanese to question US production methods. In the post-war economic struggle, a Japanese named Jehiro Ishikawa recognized that his nation must avoid repeating the same mistakes made by the United States. He assembled Japan's leading industrialists. They became convinced that their only future lay in *total quality improvement*. Ironically, Japan's company presidents founded their quality revolution through the work of two American management experts – Dr Joseph M. Juran and Dr W. Edwards Deming. The two were invited to Japan to talk to company leaders and establish the quality philosophy as a way of enabling Japan to compete in world markets. Deming started from the principle that 85% of a company's problems lay in the processes used in getting things done, and Juran completed the picture for the Japanese by stressing the customer's point of view of a product's 'fitness for use', advocating extensive training in hands-on management to provide what customers expect. The result was to eliminate anything that did not add value, and focus all processes on customers' requirements.

Companies in the United States took a further 30 years to grasp the significance of this total quality approach and regarded the success in the east as the 'Japanese miracle', attributing it to culture and consensus management. The central theme of the quality philosophy is that of continuous quality improvement. The quest for quality is and must be a continuous cycle that never ends. The ultimate goal is achieving perfection or zero defect. Deming conceptualized his approach in terms of the Deming Wheel, the basis of which is that all activities with a measurable output are processes and that perfection is the ultimate goal. See Figure 7.2.

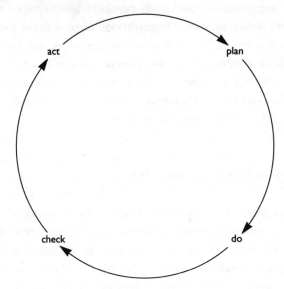

Figure 7.2: The Deming Wheel

Rising expectations of customers

What might have been acceptable 15, 5 or even 1 year ago may no longer be acceptable to today's customers and even derisory to tomorrow's. Increasingly, customers are expecting high standards in the products they buy, and raising those standards as new products and services create new norms. Those norms apply not only to the product itself, but to the whole package of services and the presentation associated with it. In most cases, where an established product has faded from the market, it has not done so because it was necessarily a poor product, but because customers' expectations had been raised by a product that fulfilled their needs better. For example, the widespread use of refrigeration has taken away most of the market for canned or bottled cream, neither of which was able to provide the same taste as fresh cream. The customer wanted the genuine taste and expressed preferences in the purchases.

Quality is defined solely by the customer. Part of the reason for the demand for quality lies in changing social patterns. People are in general more highly educated, living life at a faster pace, and will not tolerate the waste of time from products and services that do not deliver what they promise. Organizations wishing to prosper have kept up with this trend; the best have anticipated it and are ahead. The challenge to British and European organizations is whether they can benefit from the experience of the Japanese and Americans in total quality. The advantage they have is that they can short-cut their learning curve. The disadvantage is their inertia.

Quality activity in the NHS

Keyser (1989) suggests that the major problem facing NHS managers on quality is not in recognizing the need for it, but in how they make it happen. He develops this notion further by highlighting the fact that much of the progress on quality is still taking place within the professions rather than across them. Keyser's words ring true even now. However, he suggested then that if the experience of industry does have relevance, it shows that while efforts in customer organizational efficiency and quality assurance have produced good results, the excellent companies are those dedicated to total quality management (TQM). Before attempting to answer Keyser's question on relevance in the NHS attention is now drawn to those components of quality which are already receiving attention.

Patient satisfaction is a priority concern in the NHS. The NHS aims to produce services that satisfy patient needs and expectations, both efficiently and ensuring quality control and improvement. Through regional liaison, the annual review and other monitoring functions of the Department of Health (DoH), there arises the serious attention now given to the appropriateness of service delivery to the individual and the community. Other aspects of what industry might regard as marketing include patient training programmes, surveys of patient satisfaction and option appraisal applied to service quality improvement. Whether health care professionals agree or not is open to question, but there is a 'commercial' transaction between them and their patients. There is an indirect cost to patients through wasted time waiting, increased anxiety through not knowing what is going on, or the lack of control over some part of their lives. These issues can seldom be addressed by any one of the parties involved on their own.

Financial efficiency is high on the agenda of most managers in the NHS and is being tackled at the general level through improvements in planning and budgeting, resource management projects, cost-benefit studies of contracting out services like laundry, catering and cleaning as well as through income generation schemes. At the personal level, the introduction of individual performance review (IPR), and performance related pay (PRP) for senior managers, though contentious to many, are steps towards increasing efficiency. Task groups are often set up to target specific goals such as the reduction in waiting lists and inter-authority league tables have been established including for example a paper in 1988 from York University, 'Hospital deaths - the missing link; measuring outcomes in hospital data' (Kind 1988). Medical insurance claims although still not on the American scale are beginning to oblige changes in practice.

Quality assurance and standard setting

These involve the measure of service against expectations and methods of improvement. The World Health Authority aimed that by 1990 member states would have effective mechanisms for ensuring quality of patient care. This was widely recognized in the NHS and all purchasing consortia and provider units have a designated senior manager responsible for quality assurance (QA). Many subsequently produced strategy documents for QA in health care. The philosophies behind QA in health care are well developed by two key writers, Dr Robert Maxwell and Dr Avedis Donabedian.

In an article written in May 1984, Dr Robert Maxwell, Secretary to the King Edward's Fund Hospital of London, begins by stating that the concern about quality of care must be as old as medicine itself. But an honest concern about quality, however genuine, is not the same as a methodical assessment based on reliable evidence. Still less is it quality control which implies compliance with predetermined standards, as in an industrial process. There are however a number of mechanisms for assessment of quality of care in the United Kingdom including:

1   Educational accreditation for training purposes. The Royal Colleges, the Nursing Regulatory bodies, and their equivalents in other professions, all inspect the relevant departments and services provided by institutions to satisfy themselves that training arrangements in them meet the (generally rather shadowy) standards they require.

2   The confidential enquiry into maternal deaths (DoH 1986).

3   Clinical chemistry: the UK National Quality Control Scheme.

4   The Health Advisory Service and the National Development Team which have organized multi-disciplinary teams to visit the major long-stay institutions to examine standards of care, and recommend improvements when appropriate.

5   Peer review in General Practice. In 1980 the Royal College of General Practitioners set out to develop a framework defining and auditing standards of care (Board of Censors 1981).

6   Cluster analysis of performance indicators. Developed by Yates (1982) the idea of cluster analysis uses statistical data from standard sources such as the Hospital Activity Analysis.

These examples illustrate attempts to assess quality through external review. In addition medical departments have their own internal reviews as an integral part of the commitment to quality of care.

Maxwell goes on to say that no doubt the majority view amongst British doctors is that assessing and safeguarding the quality of medical care are matters best left to voluntary initiatives from consenting adults – self audit is good; external audit is a threat. Nevertheless, important as self assessment is, it is unlikely to be efficient. He goes on to suggest that there are six dimensions of health care quality:

1 access to services

2 relevance to need (for the whole community)

3 effectiveness (for individual patients)

4 equity (fairness)

5 social acceptability

6 efficiency and economy

Quality must be seen as a whole, not in fragmented parts. Maxwell concludes by saying that the last thing required is the creation of a quality assurance or quality control scheme that is insensitive to the variation, autonomy and trust implicit in health care. However, he feels it should not be beyond human wit to keep it simple, while providing a framework within which the quality of care may be studied, discussed, protected and improved. He feels that this will require encouragement, experiment and the sharing of ideas. It will call for a mixture of assessment – standards, data analysis, sampling and fellow-professional peer review and consumer opinion, tailored to an understanding of the multidimensional nature of quality itself.

Dr Avedis Donabedian (1980) recognizes that judgement of quality is not simply a technical professional matter, it also includes interpersonal aspects where consumer opinion is at least important. This links up with the emphasis in the Griffiths Report (1983) on lack of sensitivity to the consumer views in the NHS. Moreover, one of the worst aspects of recent initiatives by the Department of Health, is the persistently dreary emphasis on managerial efficiency, to the neglect of what the NHS is actually trying to achieve. It is essential that discussion about the quality of effectiveness of care be reinforced to the centre of the debate as they are, in the end, the more important dimensions of health service performance.

Donabedian's major communication on the quality of care is a claim that there was a time not too long ago when the questions of assessing quality could not have been asked. Quality of care was, he says, considered something of a mystery: real, capable of being perceived and appreciated but not subject to measurement. The very attempt to measure quality seemed then to denature and belittle it. Now, however, there is a great interest in understanding the quality of medical care and those who have not experienced the intricacies of clinical practice, demand measures that are easy, precise and complete. While some elements in the quality of care are easy to define and measure, there are still some profundities that continue to elude measurement.

Before attempting to assess quality of care, either in general terms or in any particular site or situation, Donabedian asserts that it is necessary to come to an agreement on the elements that constitute it. To proceed to measurement without a firm foundation of prior agreement on what comprises quality is to court disaster. He outlines two elements in the performance of medical practitioners, one technical, the other interpersonal. Technical performance depends on the knowledge and judgement used in arriving at the appropriate strategies of care and in implementing those strategies. The judgement in technical performance is made in comparison with the best in practice. The management of the interpersonal relationships is, he says, the second component in the practitioner's practice and is a vitally important element. Through interpersonal exchange, the patient communicates information necessary for aiming at a diagnosis, as well as preferences necessary for selecting the most appropriate methods of care. Through this exchange the clinician provides information on the nature of the illness and its management and motivates the patient to active collaboration in care. Clearly the interpersonal process is a vehicle by which technical care is implemented and on which its success depends. Notwithstanding, Donabedian points out that whilst the management of the interpersonal process is so important, it is often ignored in assessments in quality of care. There are many reasons for this: information about interpersonal process is not easily available; in the medical record, special effort is needed to obtain it. Second, the criteria and standards that permit precise measurement of the interpersonal process are not well developed, or have not been sufficiently called upon to undertake the task. It may also be because the management of the interpersonal process must adapt to so many variations in the preferences and expectations of individual patients that general guidelines do not serve sufficiently well.

Donabedian has developed a quality model which has been adopted by other practitioners as a framework against which to write standards of care. He describes an approach to the assessment of quality of care using a classification of three categories: 'structure', 'process', and 'outcome'.

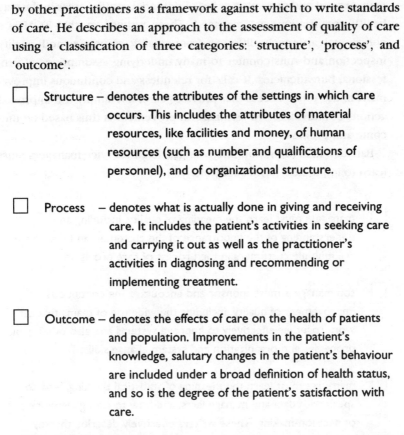

Structure – denotes the attributes of the settings in which care occurs. This includes the attributes of material resources, like facilities and money, of human resources (such as number and qualifications of personnel), and of organizational structure.

Process – denotes what is actually done in giving and receiving care. It includes the patient's activities in seeking care and carrying it out as well as the practitioner's activities in diagnosing and recommending or implementing treatment.

Outcome – denotes the effects of care on the health of patients and population. Improvements in the patient's knowledge, salutary changes in the patient's behaviour are included under a broad definition of health status, and so is the degree of the patient's satisfaction with care.

The three-part approach to quality assessment is possible only because good structure increases the likelihood of good process and good process increases the likelihood of good outcome.

Donabedian and Maxwell have made an invaluable contribution to the quality assurance process in the setting of health care. Their quality assurance models whilst designed in the context of medical practice have been widely adopted by other professionals in developing audit mechanisms and standards of practice. An attempt is now made to explore the distinction between quality assurance and TQM.

Quality, total quality and costs

In a paper published in the summer of 1990, McLaughlin and Kaluzny argue that total quality represents a total paradigm shift in health care management and presents a series of potential conflict areas in the way health organizations are managed. These writers say that TQM is a conceptual approach different from quality assurance and quality inspection and runs counter to many underlying assumptions of professional bureaucracies. It calls for relentless and continuous improvement in the total process that provides care, not simply the improved actions of individual professionals. Improvement is thus based on outcome and process.

Batalden et al (1989) outline what the health service managers must learn to implement TQM successfully:

☐ managers must learn the meaning of quality, including an understanding of the importance of the customer, and that there are multiple customers in the process of care provision;

☐ top managers must sponsor and encourage the continuous improvement of quality, including the wide use of teams that can work together effectively to improve systems and also other group processes and organization and system change skills;

☐ managers must learn the meaning of statistical thinking, how to speak with data and manage facts, and how to take guesswork out of decision-making. These writers effectively describe the key elements in the resource management projects currently under way in the NHS.

McLaughlin and Kaluzny go on to say that TQM demands that change be based on the needs of the customer, not the values of the providers. It requires the meaningful participation of all personnel and a rapid and thoughtful response from top managers to suggestions made by participating personnel. Managers are no longer able to stifle the suggestions of personnel by requiring that all decisions be reviewed at a higher level.

TQM is more than a change in values and responsiveness by top management. It requires rigorous process flow and statistical analysis, evaluation of all ongoing activities, and the recognition and application of underlying principles affecting individuals and groups within an organization. It requires accepting the fundamental assumption that most problems encountered in an organization are the result not of errors by administrative or clinical professionals, but the inability of the structure - within which all personnel function - to perform adequately.

An obvious conflict is between the relentless inquiry of TQM and the established norms of professional autonomy. This is not merely a conflict between managers and clinical professionals. It is a fundamental challenge to the way all professionals think about quality, evaluate and regulate themselves, and gain and protect their professional domains and autonomy. TQM does not respect existing professional standards, it is continually demanding new ones.

Finally, TQM challenges the prevailing model of who is the customer. The customer in TQM is not only the patient, but also the many users of a department's output, as has already been observed. Again, the criterion is not whether the work meets professional standards, but whether the user, often a member of another profession, is satisfied with its timeliness and utility.

The reality is that both models - TQM and the professional bureaucracy - must be accommodated if TQM is to make a difference in health care organizations. For example, Galbraith (1973) outlines the importance of the professional model in handling the flood of technical information that medical and nursing research has developed. He suggests that specialization is a way of handling information overload, especially in the absence of other information: processing alternatives such as a common management information system or lateral linkages for information co-ordination. In fact, one can see TQM as a methodology for developing lateral linkages in the health care organization that transfer information between disciplines as needed. It is a powerful method of lateral technology transfer in a traditionally highly compartmentalized organization.

Conflicts between the two models

The nature of the organizational change required to implement TQM can be outlined by contrasting the two models and evaluating the points of conflict (see Figure 7.3). Whilst they are not mutually

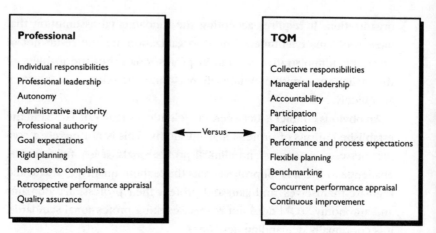

Professional		TQM
Individual responsibilities		Collective responsibilities
Professional leadership		Managerial leadership
Autonomy		Accountability
Administrative authority		Participation
Professional authority	◄—Versus—►	Participation
Goal expectations		Performance and process expectations
Rigid planning		Flexible planning
Response to complaints		Benchmarking
Retrospective performance appraisal		Concurrent performance appraisal
Quality assurance		Continuous improvement

Figure 7.3: Areas of conflict between two organizational models

exclusive and whilst the observed points of conflict will vary between organizations, each of the models requires explicit recognition.

Whilst the debate around the professional role culture and the managerial task culture in the TQM context may continue, Scott (1990) argues that the pursuit of quality management embraces all the initiatives being developed in the NHS at present, e.g. clinical audit, which itself embraces medical audit and quality improvement. This, Scott says, has to be the most effective way to ensure that care of an appropriate cost is delivered. Therefore, managing quality controls costs. Scott supports his argument by saying that terms like 'quality' and 'outcome' have attracted considerable academic literature. They are particularly hard to define in health care as they have many different dimensions and for example, those things that are most important to the patient may only be one aspect of the quality of care as seen by the clinician. Although it might be difficult to measure quality, it is much easier to agree on what constitutes 'bad quality care'. Many people will be familiar with the sort of complaint that involves a thorough review of the medical files. It is often found that a patient's reluctance to complain has finally been overcome by a build up of relatively minor, yet significant failings. A long wait in a casualty department, surly or uncommunicative staff, iatrogenic events and complications are often part of a sorry list. It is easy to see how each element can be tackled but quite often the totality springs from a lack of corporate commitment to quality as well as a lack of multidisciplinary working.

Borrowing from the 'quality' literature Scott continues to say that 'getting it right first time' is a well known slogan in TQM programmes. Because of its origin in the manufacturing industries there is often scepticism about its application in the health environment. After all, in a car factory, it is clear what mistakes in a spot weld or paint spray will cost in terms of materials and to see the need to put the defects right, and, that if a little more care and attention even at the expense of some time can result in less or even zero defects, then it will be cost effective.

However, harassed clinicians already working under considerable pressure are not always assured that this sort of motor industry thinking is appropriate in hospitals. That said, who bears the cost of getting it wrong has got to be a concern. If a clerical error results in a patient having an x-ray without notes, the fact that she has to re-attend subsequently is a source of irritation to the x-ray department and will certainly carry a cost; but far more importantly it means the patient will have to spend more time in hospital than she might otherwise. The cost to the patient and family is hard to measure but, quite apart from the need to return patients to their home environment as soon as practical, in order to relieve psychological stress, the chance of postoperative complication for example is reduced by short stay. Clearly, although some costs are material and are born within the hospital, the overall impact on the patient of getting things wrong is a key issue. As John Ruskin said 'getting it right is better than putting it right'.

Although it is suggested that getting things right first time will reduce costs, there is no suggestion that high quality medicine is always low cost. Setting standards for the treatment of patients and monitoring against those standards implies that certain costs are associated with certain levels of quality. For example, it may be agreed policy locally that all concussed patients exhibiting certain symptoms should have a CT scan. Other hospitals might adopt different criteria which result in less patients receiving a scan. Effectively this is defining a level of quality and its associated costs. There is no suggestion that one is necessarily more appropriate than the other and standards must be set locally by staff themselves. What is being suggested is that managing the quality of care in effect manages the cost of care. Providing it is ensured that patients are treated in the way the clinicians had determined in advance, then the cost of care is managed at the same time.

Deming supports the quality cost debate in postulating 'Good quality does not necessarily mean high quality. It means a degree of uniformity and dependability at low cost with a quality suited to the market' Walton (1989).

The first barrier in attempting to create a strategic focus on quality in the NHS is that most people have a blurred idea about what 'quality' is. They typically equate quality with expense – a Rolex watch or Wedgwood china. It is possible to pay a high price for an inferior product or service. It is not rare to find highly priced restaurants that do not always provide excellent food and service. Equally it is possible to pay relatively little for high quality, for example, for Marks and Spencer clothes.

Another common confusion is between good quality and high quality. Processes such as dialysis need 'high quality' water, i.e., a high grade of water from which impurities have been reduced down to levels of a few parts per million or less. For most industrial purposes, however, 'good quality' tap water is perfectly adequate, and indeed would probably be regarded as high quality. Much the same comparison can be made with nurse staffing levels. It is not uncommon to hear nurses argue that levels of staff equate with levels of quality of nursing care. Without any tangible service specification of standards of conformity, such a claim is invalid. The Resource Management Project has challenged nurses to conduct analyses of workload, examine skill mix and set standards, It is a dangerous misconception that achieving quality is too expensive to be justified. The traditional view assumes that beyond a certain point, investing in quality becomes subject to the law of eliminating all errors, deviations from requirements and that inconsistencies cannot be justified by the savings made. Such a view fails to see quality as a strategic issue and fails to understand that the costs of quality are much wider than scrap and reworking. The opportunity to integrate quality of care consideration, dialogue and the effective management of resources deserves to be exploited.

CONCLUSION

It is suggested that managers are faced with two sets of problems – those of today and those of tomorrow. The problems of today concern the immediate needs of the organization; how to maintain quality, how to manage within budgets, employment issues, service provision, public relations and so on. The tendency could be to dwell on such problems, without adequate attention to the future. In the NHS, those organizations where quality is being addressed now are planning a future, because they are developing plans and methods to stay in a competitive market. The next and final chapter discusses the concept of marketing in health care. The old adage 'the customer is always right' used to be a phrase reserved for salespeople at retail counters. Today, the NHS is finding that it has a new meaning as consumer attitudes (whether the consumer be the purchasers of health care or indeed the patient or client) help shape the marketplace.

ACTION GUIDELINES

The following guidelines will help you consider some of the quality issues discussed in the chapter and apply them to your clinical service:

1 **Consider the issue of 'quality' in the NHS today**

☐ **how is quality measured in your work area?**

☐ **list five elements of a 'quality service'**

2 **Consider the perspectives of quality in the NHS**

☐ **who are the users of your service?**

☐ **who are the providers?**

☐ **who are the purchasers?**

3 **Consider quality management in your organization**

☐ **what quality systems are in place?**

☐   list five examples where you believe
      improvement is possible.

☐   how are you managing quality to control
      costs?

4   Identify a quality initiative that you could lead

☐   what is the status quo?

☐   what needs to be done?

☐   what are your communication networks?

☐   what method of assessment would you use
      as success criteria?

REFERENCES

Batalden P et al (1989) Quality improvement: the role and application of research methods *The Journal of Health Administration Education* **7**(3): 577–583.

Board of Censors, Royal College of General Practitioners (1981) What sort of doctor? *Journal of the Royal College of General Practitioners.* **31**: 698–702.

DoH (1986) *Confidential Enquiry into Maternal Deaths in England and Wales, 1979–81.* London: HMSO.

Donabedian A (1980) *The Definition of Quality and Approaches to its Assessment.* Ann Arbor, Michigan: Health Administration Press.

Galbraith J (1973) *Designing Complex Organisations.* Reading, MA: Addison-Wesley.

Griffiths R (1983) *NHS Management Inquiry. Griffiths Report.* London: DHSS.

Handy C (1990) *The Age of Unreason*. London: Arrow Books Ltd.

Keyser W (1989) Healthcare, is TQ relevant? *Total Quality Management*, February.

Kind P (1988) *Hospital Deaths — The Missing Link: Measuring Outcomes in Hospital Data*. York University.

Major J (1991) *The Citizen's Charter 'Raising the Standards'*. London: HMSO.

McLaughlin C P and Kaluzny A D (1990) Total quality management in health: making it work *Healthcare Management Review* **IS(3)**: 7–14.

Maxwell R (1984) Perspectives in NHS management: Quality assessment in health *British Medical Journal* **288**: 1470–1472.

Scott T (1990) *Managing Quality to Control Costs. Resource Management: The Leading Edge*. London: Resource Management Unit, DoH.

Walton M (1989) *The Deming Management Method*. Mercury Business Books.

Yates J (1982) *Hospital beds*. London: Heinemann.

FURTHER READING

☐ Crosby P B (1979) *Quality is Free*. Maidenhead: McGraw-Hill.

☐ Major J (1991) *Citizen's Charter and Patient's Charter*. London: HMSO.

☐ Peters T and Austen N *A Passion for Excellence*. London: Fontana Collins.

MARKETING AND HEALTH CARE

8

It has been frequently stated that there is much scope within the NHS for improvement in the delivery, quality and choice of service provision. The lack of response to consumer preferences has been a major criticism of health services in recent years as the public's expectations of, and demand for, health services become much more explicit.

CHAPTER AIMS

☐ To outline the role of marketing in health care management in the context of the current NHS reforms

☐ To apply some basic marketing concepts and techniques to clinical practice and management

CONTEXT

The NHS reforms (DoH 1991) have been seen as a logical extension of the 'new public health' process, which looks at whole and minority populations, assessing the public's health and health care needs. Many of the changes to the NHS have helped to begin a shift in emphasis from a hospital to a patient-led service. This ensures that it is the patient or client rather than the organization that is central to all work. This is expressed particularly in the developments of integration in primary, secondary and social care, with many health care professionals developing partnerships and working collaboratively with other sectors. Examples are social services, police, voluntary and commercial organizations. The process of health needs assessment will begin to challenge the appropriateness of current services and provide a framework for future development.

Purchasing health care

The objective of purchasing has been first, to ensure the integration of care services, second, to achieve the most efficient and effective deployment of resources across the primary and secondary care sectors, and thirdly, to make the NHS work in the best way it can to support the local population. The role of the District Health Authorities (DHAs) and Family Health Service Authorities (FHSAs) in preventing ill health and securing health care for their residents provides the main focus for this work. The separation of the purchaser and provider roles in health care is perhaps one of the most radical developments as yet encountered in the NHS's history, and it is this separation that is central to the success or failure of the NHS reforms. To achieve a purchasing role, responsibility for the funding and provision of services has been separated with the introduction of NHS contracts or service agreements which are to be negotiated between purchasers and providers of health care (see Figure 8.1). As purchasers, the primary responsibilities of DHAs will be to ensure that, within the available resources, services are secured through the contracting process to meet the health care needs of their resident populations. General Practitioner Fundholders (GPFH) have become purchasers and are at

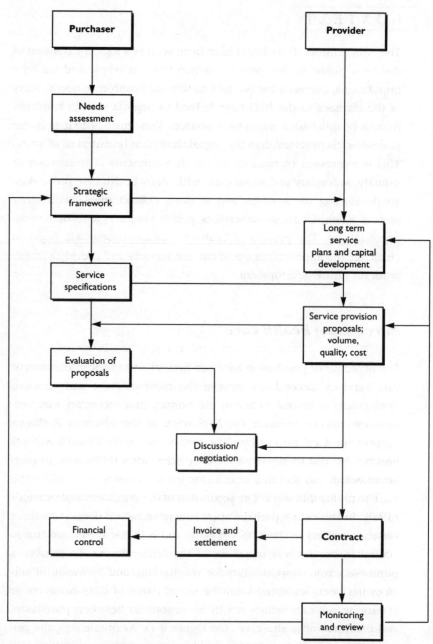

Figure 8.1: The contracting process. From Healthcare Financial Management
Association (1991)

present responsible for a budget to purchase a range of non-emergency health treatments, prescribing expenditure, part of the costs of the practice staff and from April 1993 community nursing services, in terms of health visiting and district nursing. Unlike commercial organizations, the procurement and provision of health care is, on the whole, a collaborative venture between the purchaser and provider to ensure that health care goals are reached, with the overall responsibility of 'fair play' lying with Regional Health Authorities and ultimately the Department of Health.

Providing health care

The provider role necessitates providers of health care services delivering contracted services within quality and quantity specifications to one or a number of purchasers, in return for agreed charges. The provider units will in the main be either directly managed units (of DHAs) or NHS Trust units (directly responsible to the NHS management executive). However, this will largely depend on the effectiveness of those services delivered by the NHS. It is becoming increasingly apparent that there are many non-NHS agencies that have experience in providing health care services, for example, health promotion and counselling services. Purchasers, therefore are looking to provide cost effective, patient responsive services. Should a non-NHS agency be able to deliver a better service, then that option must be considered.

The philosophy for the reforms, it is said, continues to embrace the 1948 principles for the NHS, that is, comprehensiveness, equality of access and largely free at the point of use. The added element of competition, as it is anticipated, will serve to improve the effectiveness and efficiency of health care delivery. This should result from the improvements in value for money expected from arrangements for commissioning care services such as detailed service specifications and business planning. Increased competition between service providers, should lead to improved quality and reduced costs, as providers assess more closely the processes, outputs and outcomes of service delivery. Increased emphasis on the appropriateness, accessibility, range and balance of services to be provided should enable consumer-responsive services to be developed, which will more closely match the needs and preferences of service users.

The idea of introducing market forces into the NHS environment was first documented in 1985 by Professor A Enthoven, an American health economist. When presenting a review of some of the problems of the organization and management in the NHS, Enthoven introduced the concept of an 'internal market model', recommending that a DHA should resemble a nationalized company. It would buy and sell services from and to other DHAs and trade with the private sector. Enthoven also noted that whilst the NHS commanded widespread support, it provided few incentives for efficiency and there appeared to be wide variation in practice, with little attention to health outcomes (Enthoven 1985). Prior to Enthoven's *Reflections on the NHS*, Sir Roy Griffiths (1983) was commissioned to advise the Government on 'the effective and efficient use and management of manpower and related resources' in the NHS. This report made recommendations that strong local general management must be developed, and that clinicians must be encouraged to become involved in the management process. The NHS reforms build on both of these recommendations, and it has been the separation between the purchase of health care and its provision, with the central aim of resources following patients, that has secured the development of a 'market' environment. The purchasers of health care services have assumed a customer role and patients a consumer role.

To understand the principles of marketing and its use for clinical managers, it would be useful first of all to outline commercial marketing principles and then to discuss the transposability of those principles to health care.

Commercial marketing

Commercial marketing today has evolved from a production-orientated approach to a customer-orientated approach. A production-orientated approach focused on organizing a company's resources to produce and sell its products. Today's marketing concepts call for a reorientation of the company's way of conducting its business. Instead of trying to get customers to buy what the company produced, a marketing-orientated company would try to sell what the customer wanted. It is, therefore, a misconception to describe the marketing concept as the advertising and selling of goods, it is much broader, involving extensive market research and strategic planning, with a primary focus to increase consumer responsiveness. (It is important to stress this point, as many health care professionals' view of marketing is purely the advertising and selling of goods. Hence a distrust has developed of the role of marketing in health care.) Cavusgil describes marketing as ' . . . a bridge, linking the organisation with its environment, orientating it towards customers and other constituencies, and helping management to position its efforts in relation to those of its competitors' (Cavusgil 1986).

Because of the historical, production-orientated approach to marketing, the introduction of the marketing concept has required a number of changes within commercial organizations. These have principally been in management attitudes, organization structure and management methods and procedures. The overriding aim is to ensure that the company's internal activities and utilization of its resources are organized to meet and satisfy the needs of its customers.

Commercial organizations operate in a highly competitive environment and need to keep a competitive edge on their rivals to remain successful. Companies exist to conduct business and the business environment is the 'market'. A market is the demand for a product or service. Before a company develops a product or service, it must first identify consumer demand, otherwise resources invested in product development could be wasted. The prime objective, therefore, is to establish what the consumers want and what price they are prepared to pay. This is achieved through the use of robust marketing techniques. These techniques will be used to a greater or lesser degree depending on the size and complexity of the organization, product and market.

Marketing techniques

Marketing techniques underpin decisions related to investment in product development and market penetration. The marketing technique that is critical to the success or failure of the product and from which all other techniques are informed is market research. This provides a comprehensive analysis of the market environment through the systematic and objective review of the facts relating to the product, that is, its market, competitors, consumer needs, wants, demands, and many other factors that impact on the product's development. This valuable information enables companies to develop market strategy and marketing mix (design and characteristics of the service). This in turn determines resource allocation with regard to the business plan, and analysis of environmental factors through the use of a marketing audit. Marketing audit seeks to analyse the organization's strengths and weaknesses in relation to marketing, and the opportunities and threats that the market provides for the organization: this analysis establishes a profile of the business and its capabilities in relation to those of its competitors. If a marketing audit is properly completed it will form the basis for setting realistic marketing objectives, goals and strategies. The audit will support the development of the strategy determining where effort is to be placed, which markets it chooses to penetrate and what types of service or product it will attempt to provide for those markets. An essential element of any market strategy is the marketing mix, this refers to the combination of variable elements that make up the design of a product or service. This is commonly achieved through the application of a model to determine the most effective delivery method of a product or service to the customer. For commercial marketing, McCarthy used a model called the 'Four Ps' which describes: *product, place, promotion* and *price* (McCarthy 1978). These are used to determine what the customer wants, where it can be obtained, when and how it can be obtained and how the product is priced. This model will be supported by extensive market research.

The development of the product will impact on the rest of the marketing mix. For example, if the product does not satisfy customer needs then no matter what resources are allocated to the place, promotion and price aspects of the marketing mix, the product will fail. The product is not an end in itself, but encompasses the process from conception, through development to completion, and continuing with ongoing product research and development. As the central aim of marketing is to help the organization remain viable and achieve continuous growth, the marketing mix of the service must be carefully developed. The placing of the product or service is concerned with all the problems, functions and channels involved in the manufacture and distribution of the right product to the right place, at the right time and to the right customer. Promotion is defined as the development of persuasive communications. The main tools are advertising, personal selling, sales promotion, public relations and word of mouth. Price is an important element to make the product as attractive as possible. In setting a price, the nature of the competition, customer reaction, and anticipated product performance must be taken into account to ensure an acceptable competitive price is set.

Service marketing

Health care organizations are engaged in the production of services. Production and consumption occur together. In service marketing an extended model to the Four Ps is often used to determine a more comprehensive marketing mix. These are: *people, physical evidence* and *process*. The people element is essential. Using its members, an organization needs to communicate effectively both internally between staff groups, and externally between staff and actual and potential customers; the organization must learn how to communicate the quality of its service if it is to become competitive. The external effectiveness of the communication process is also an integral part of the promotional aspects of the marketing mix. Human resource development is of paramount importance, staff training in customer relations is particularly necessary to ensure a customer responsive service. To recruit and retain high calibre staff, service organizations now more than ever before are investing in staff as their key resource, acknowledging that the staff–customer interface is critical to the reputation of the organization. Physical evidence focuses on the environment, for example, safety, atmosphere, facilities and cleanliness. Many health care organizations use external consultants and service users to advise on the physical environment. The end products that an organization will obtain are determined by the processes it uses, that is, the activities of the service. To ensure that the services are customer-orientated it is essential to involve customers (actual and potential) in its design and evaluation. The use of user groups, questionnaires, simple complaints procedures and so on provides a wealth of information to use as a focus for service development.

Health care marketing

The primary focus on marketing in organizations has been placed on business firms which typically have profit as their main objective for the business's survival. In the health care context, marketing involves an understanding of what the customers (purchasers) and consumers (patients/clients) need and demand in terms of health care, identifying the appropriate services to be offered and providing them efficiently and effectively. Marketing and quality have much in common – they both focus on the consumer and their requirements, rather than being product or service led. Private health care organizations function differently from the publicly funded NHS, in that they address a given and anticipated demand. The NHS must, on behalf of its public, address both the needs and demands of the nation's health. The 'business' of health care is the provision of comprehensive services, ensuring equality of access and in the main, providing the services free at the point of delivery.

Marketing in health care is neither new nor revolutionary in many health care systems. The USA has used marketing as a general management function for many years and in this country, private health care organizations have used marketing techniques as part of an overall business strategy. With recent trends towards greater productivity and an increasing focus on resource management and continuous quality improvement, purchasers are looking to obtain maximum quality and quantity of service from their finite purchasing resources. It is anticipated that competition will naturally develop as purchasers seek value for money services and as providers need to become competitive to secure contractual agreements and so remain viable.

As most health care provision in Britain is funded through taxation, how the organization can and ought to market will be influenced by external regulators (the Government, purchasers, Regional Health Authorities and the Department of Health), and if a hospital wishes to discontinue what it sees as an unattractive service, it will be unable to do so, if it is deemed as necessary by its regulators.

The new internal market is expected to behave in a very different way to the commercial market, since health care has different priorities and multiple objectives. The gap between supply and demand will continue to grow rather than fall, as recent trends show that by

2016 there will be an increase of about 1,785,000 people in England, of whom no fewer than 440,000 will be over 85 years of age (DoH 1991). In this situation the critics argue that marketing services will create unnecessary demand, which will continue to remain unmet, and using already limited resources to increase the demand further is not justi-fied. Advocates of marketing in health care, on the other hand, argue that marketing leads to increased consumer satisfaction and a better understanding of consumer needs through techniques such as market research and interactive marketing which help clinicians and managers develop consumer-responsive services, which form an essential part of continuous quality improvement programmes.

Transposing marketing techniques to health care

The fundamental changes discussed by marketing experts in transpos-ing orthodox commercial methods to health care is the need to have a comprehensive understanding of the NHS's health care philosophy, its objectives, publics, customers and consumers, and its values and tradi-tions; all of which are very different in many respects from commercial organizations.

There are a number of factors in marketing health care that are particular to public health care organizations that are not in the main experienced in the commercial sector:

☐ the service is not wanted (people do not want to be ill)

☐ use of the service is seldom planned

☐ consumers do not usually shop for health care as they do for other products (it is purchased on their behalf)

☐ there is limited marketing expertise and experience in the service

With the internal market in its infancy, purchasers are more likely to purchase health care from local provider units and so those units that are easily accessible to local populations (the natural catchment area) will tend to have a high market share (market share is defined as the percentage of demand being met by the provider's facilities). There will be little competition from other provider units unless the service required is not offered, only a limited range of services are available or the service is unattractive compared to the competition. Whilst there is a lack of overt competition by health services, coupled with the 'reluctant' demand placed on the service by consumers, this will to some extent impact on the necessity and usefulness of marketing techniques in health care. However, it is generally accepted that many of the service marketing techniques will provide exciting opportunities for achieving service developments and consumer reponsiveness.

Health care publics

The health care market is much larger and more complicated than its commercial counterpart. A commercial market has one main public, the consumer. A health care organization on the other hand has two main publics, the customer and the consumer. It also has a number of other publics, for example, professionals, non-fundholding GPs, pressure groups, regulatory bodies, patients' families and carers, social services etc. These various publics, particularly the regulatory bodies may in fact limit the organization's choice of market strategy and may also influence service policy. Whilst commercial organizations determine their own marketing strategy, they too will be influenced by public opinion when developing the product policy. For example, there are increasing numbers of companies developing biodegradable and natural products, as increasing numbers of the public become concerned with the destruction of the environment.

Market strategy

In the NHS a market strategy must provide the organization with the flexibility to respond quickly to consumer wishes and needs and to enable alternative patterns of service to develop, ensuring that innovation and a personalization of the service takes place (see Figure 8.2). Such innovation can already be demonstrated by the increasing interest in established Scandinavian developments, for example, hotel services, with many obstetric and gynaecology units looking to develop these services to provide a more relaxed and personal approach to health care delivery. There are also many examples of new services managed by nurses, midwives and health visitors, providing drop-in facilities, assessment clinics and specialist advice, developed as a result of patient surveys and service uptake information using basic market research techniques for improving the acceptability and appropriateness of certain services.

In developing any strategy, identifying the organization's objectives is the basis for all future work. Although business organizations have multiple objectives they tend to be dominated by one main objective – the drive for profit maximization, with little thought for the consumer after the commodity has been purchased, with the exception of after sales service, where the product is faulty or requires servicing. Health care is very different in this respect. It aims to provide benefit to the consumer and to prevent demand for the service through the promotion of good health and the prevention of ill health and where illness is established, providing treatment, rehabilitation and if necessary, continuing and terminal care services. There may, because of ever

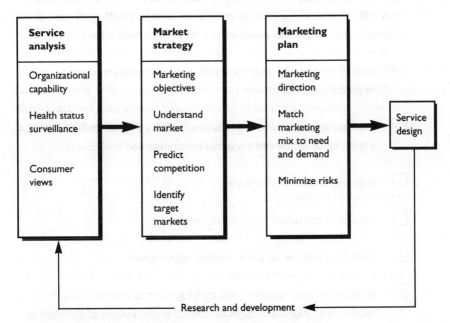

Figure 8.2: Marketing process for service development

increasing demand for services, need to be a move toward 'demarketing' methods (used to reduce the demand for the service), to allow more needs-based rather than demand-based services to be developed. A target for this type of marketing (which is unique to public sector health care organizations), would be so-called fashionable treatments that have no demonstrable health gain benefits to consumers, for example, some types of cosmetic surgery.

The NHS pursues several key objectives at the same time; these objectives are different to private health care and commercial organizations, as both the purchasers and providers strive to address international, national and local health care objectives. International objectives support the World Health Organization's strategy – Health for All by the Year 2000, national objectives encompass the NHS reforms and Community Care Act, the Health of the Nation White Paper, and the Patient's Charter. Locally owned provider objectives may, for example, involve the development of cardiovascular services, or a need to attract specialist skills for paediatric and theatre services. All these objectives must be considered when developing market strategy. A provider's market strategy will be targeted at the two primary segments (segmentation identifies target markets): routine and specialist services, and a number of customer groups (staff, patients, GPs, hospital consultants and purchasers). Key marketing aims will be to:

- [ ] ensure marketing concepts are integral to the health care organization's objectives;

- [ ] raise awareness of the organization, its full range of services and expertise to actual and potential customers and consumers;

- [ ] improve market performance;

- [ ] develop a consumer-responsive service;

- [ ] develop a reputation for a 'leading edge' service;

- [ ] provide ongoing research and development to inform changes in market conditions and facilitate the continual review of the market strategy, and in so doing, enhance service development

Competition will be on a different basis within each segment. Elective and day case admissions are commercially attractive as they are controllable. Emergency services on the other hand are not. Whilst in a commercial sense the obvious segment to penetrate would be the elective services (as do private health care organizations), the challenge to the NHS is to provide a comprehensive and equitable service to consumers, and to ensure that the less attractive (in marketing terms) services are available. The purchasers of health care identify them as 'core services', purchasing these services through the contracting arrangements. Further segmentation takes place within service agreements based on criteria for grouping consumers, for example, specialty services, geographical location, care groups etc. The identification of niche markets (a target market where there is little or no competition) will be attractive to units with specialist or unique services for example, neurology, nephrology, homeopathy and other alternative therapies, as these services in particular will be able to take advantage of extra contractual referrals (and the income they bring) to further service development.

Marketing audit

Marketing audit techniques using SWOT analysis will provide a useful framework for identifying service and business development opportunities, for example, to defend existing services, expand core services, and identify possible diversification of present services. It is essential to define the health market, determining its size, trends, influencing factors (external and internal), its segments by geography and patient, the present market share, competitors and the scope for developing niche markets. The audit must also take into consideration consumer characteristics, for example, who uses the present service, profiling current and potential patients by age, sex, where they live and their social class (to determine public health consequences). It is important also to consider the patients' needs in relation to the services provided and the patients' attitudes to current provision. An objective review of current services will provide vital information for service development and a number of questions need to be asked, for example:

☐ is the service accessible/acceptable?

☐ does it have all the necessary features and are the patient's needs met?

☐ how are the services used?

☐ is the service relevant to the need of the whole community?

☐ is the service effective in achieving its aims?

☐ where do the services stand in relation to those of competitors?

☐ what would the market potential be for a new service?

☐ do any of the services have a low or decreasing demand or are out of date and if so what measures are being taken to address this?

The review must incorporate the views of both users and providers of the service. To undertake a comprehensive marketing audit the organization needs to develop an understanding of public health, the purchaser's responsibilities for the public's health, the consumer's needs and its competitor's capabilities.

Market research

The use of robust market research techniques applicable to health care must be developed by both the purchasers and providers, to facilitate the purchasing and provision of services that adequately reflect the population's need, and a reappraisal of those services that have been historically delivered. Health care demands analysis of all populations (minority as well as majority populations), and their characteristics, for example, migration, social factors, morbidity and mortality, personal and popular opinions, all require careful analysis. It is essential, if a consumer-responsive service is to be developed, that research is conducted into patients' needs for health care. With relatively little information available describing needs and preferences, the sharing of information between purchasers, providers and other agencies must be considered. At present information for market research is obtained from published sources, i.e. population trends, economic trends, social trends, census and public health reports, performance measures (covering almost every activity and service), and GP referral patterns. Accurate, comprehensive information of patient 'careers' through the health service is limited. Analysis techniques when established will provide information, not only for the planning and forecasting of service provision, but also for the monitoring and evaluation of health care processes and outcomes.

A marketing mix in health care

THE PRODUCT

Health is a fundamental human right. Health is a vital resource to the individual, the community and society as a whole. Health care needs to be sensitive to the wider concept of health rather than to traditional attitudes that have focused on illness. Health care provision is multi-faceted, it is diverse and complex, it is essentially intangible and the services in the main are produced at the time they are being consumed. Health care is influenced by ethical, political, economical, social and technological factors. Because of its social and ethical factors it is seen as a 'public good' and so finds itself under constant public scrutiny and the focus of continuous political and public debate. Public scrutiny is much more of a consideration for health care organizations as they are expected to operate in the public interest, so too are their marketing activities.

Aspects of the product

☐ characteristics of the service

☐ strengths and weaknesses of the service and its provision

☐ does the service meet the needs and preferences of purchasers and consumers?

☐ how is it better and/or different from competing services?

☐ how is service quality defined by professionals/purchasers/consumers?

☐ control mechanisms to monitor, review and evaluate service provision

☐ service design and performance in relation to local and corporate objectives, business plan targets and service agreements

PROMOTION

The promotion of services is at present seen by many professionals as unethical and threatening, whereas in the commercial market, aggressive promotion campaigns are seen as an essential tool to ensure that the customers purchase the product. Promotion of health care needs to be sensitive and carefully monitored: glossy brochures, videos and gimmicky promotion may well be seen as a waste of limited resources, both internally, if a particular specialty has been refused additional resources and externally, if consumers are experiencing excessive waiting times for admission. Health promotion is a key task for all health care workers and because of this, many professionals advise their consumers against using many commercial organizations' products. This is referred to as 'anti-marketing', and prime examples are advice related to smoking, alcohol consumption and diet. As Sheaff points out, 'anti-marketing is a necessary part of health promotion; it will be unpopular with the marketing and advertising establishments but these are not strongly placed to complain about unethical methods.' (Sheaff 1991) It can be beneficial to involve the public in using marketing techniques, such as 'social marketing'. In using this method it is possible to encourage the local and national media to 'advertise' good news stories, innovation in the organization, capital developments and health promotion campaigns. For example, Mr X receives the first heart transplant in Liverpool, alternative therapies are now available at Trust hospital X, hospital Y builds crèche facilities. Not only will this raise the local and national health care profile within the community, it fosters an ownership by the public of health and health related issues. Although this type of marketing is free, it has the disadvantage of less control over what is being marketed – the publicity may not always be good! This form of marketing is particularly acceptable to many members of the health care organizations and is increasingly being used to enhance income generation ventures within the service. There is also a trend for health care organizations to capitalize on other organizations to help raise extra funding. This is known as 'donor marketing' and has been used by many hospitals who have a particular empathy with the public, for example children's hospitals using appeals to raise funds for equipment and toys.

Aspects of promotion

☐   image of the service you need or want to portray and to whom

☐   determining promotional media available, its usefulness and cost

☐   public relations

☐   developing persuasive communications internally and externally

THE PLACE

The place where services are delivered (location, accessibility and mobility) will of course be paramount to attract consumers. Whereas businesses can relocate or increase their outlets to penetrate a particular market segment, the NHS is severely restricted, with a tradition of consumers going to the organization, rather than the organization going to the consumer (with the exception of community and primary care). There is, however, evidence of increasing mobility in the pursuit of effectiveness, for example, the use of mobile breast screening units and operating theatres. There is also increasing demand for hospital consultants to carry out clinics at the local GP surgery, providing consumers with shorter waiting times and a service delivered in familiar surroundings near the home and possibly with access to other drop-in services (baby clinics etc.) during the visit. The primary health care team also benefits, as case discussion can take place informally between the consultant and members of the primary health care team.

As more GPs become Fundholders it is anticipated that an increasing emphasis will be placed on these types of services.

Aspects of place

☐ planning of service location

☐ accessibility of the service

☐ availability and flexibility of the service

THE PRICE

In commercial marketing, pricing the product correctly is essential to the survival of the business; whilst the NHS does not have a profit motive, it is of course concerned with the control of its expenditure. Pricing in the NHS was not seen as a priority until the implementation of the contracting process, despite a number of attempts by the Government to involve managers and clinicians in management budgeting. Resource management, when implementation is complete, aims to provide health care organizations with better financial and patient-based information. The lack of good costing information at present makes it difficult to develop competitive pricing strategies. Realistic costing and pricing in the NHS is now seen as fundamental. For contractual income, prices have initially been set on the basis of broad average specialty costs; pricing in future years is expected to see the development of more refined costing methods to reflect demand more closely. As costing information develops competitive pricing will be the goal of all provider units, as purchasers insist on a value for money service. Interestingly, while the purchasers carry the cost of health care provision, it is the consumer that experiences the quality of that provision, and the consumer's perception of quality may be very different from that of the purchaser!

Aspects of price

☐ effective and efficient management of resources

☐ demand for service

☐ realistic costing and pricing methods

☐ competitive pricing strategies

☐ purchasers' and consumers' perceived value

SERVICE DELIVERY (PEOPLE, PROCESS AND PHYSICAL EVIDENCE)

Service delivery in health care organizations is inseparable from its people (staff performing the service). Development of staff has not been a priority of the NHS, whereas in commercial service organizations staff have been seen as the company's main asset and have been developed as such. Development of staff takes time and so costs money, and as a consequence of this, the NHS has only recently accepted that it has a responsibility for its key resource – its people. In marketing a health service, the patient's judgement as to whether or not the service was good is not necessarily made on the clinical expertise that was provided, as a patient or relative may not be able to distinguish between 'good' and 'bad' care. As research now shows, judgements are often made on more intangible evidence, for example, staff attitudes, the environment, waiting times and consumers' experiences with the organization. It is important, therefore, to ensure that the consumer is integrated into the health care process: 'interactive marketing' can be used to assist this integration. Interactive techniques have already been developed in particular specialties, for example, orthopaedics and paediatrics, where many units are developing patient 'user groups' to help health care professionals and general managers identify areas of dissatisfaction and to suggest further developments to enhance the satisfaction of users of the service. This method can also be used within the organization itself, as employees have many entrepreneurial ideas on how to improve the service. Quality circles, management development programmes and staff suggestion boxes have been the initial focus for this work, and through this method the organization demonstrates its commitment to satisfying internal as well as external consumers.

The flexibility of the service can also be assessed through marketing techniques which will begin to challenge professional values, traditions and practices; these challenges may well cause conflict for clinicians and managers within the organization. Clinicians by virtue of the intimate relationship they share with their patients, must be able to adapt quickly to meet changes in consumer needs and preferences, and are well positioned to take advantage of service development opportunities as they arise. For example, market research and interactive marketing may identify a consumer demand for developments such as open visiting, clinics and day case surgery at the weekend, consultant rather than junior medical staff consultations or a preference for a midwife rather than an obstetrician-managed service. To date many of the service improvements pursued by purchasers have focused on the environment of care, that is, waiting times, patient facilities and the structural aspects of service delivery. In time, patient-based information will provide a focus for the monitoring and evaluation of the processes and outcomes of clinical care through the use of clinical audit, protocols and care profiles.

Aspects of service delivery

Process

- [ ] effectiveness of policies/procedures/practices

- [ ] management structures and processes that support service delivery

- [ ] control mechanisms to ensure that processes, outputs and outcomes are monitored, reviewed and evaluated

- [ ] action to minimize risks and optimize good practice

People

- [ ] human resource development

- [ ] consumer-orientated service (internal and external consumers)

- [ ] good communication strategies

Physical evidence

☐ adequate facilities

☐ acceptable environment for staff and consumers

☐ quality of goods

☐ tangible indicators

Stakeholders

In developing a commercial market strategy and agreeing other marketing techniques to be used in a commercial organization, there are a relatively small number of 'stakeholders' with whom to reach agreement, whereas in the NHS, with the devolution of managerial responsibility to selected clinicians through the development of clinical management teams, the number of stakeholders in the health care organization are vast, with the use of horizontal as well as vertical management structures. There are, therefore, clinicians, clinical managers and general managers to whom the strategy needs to be sold. As units develop market strategies, conflict between professional autonomy and managerial effectiveness is certain to become one of the key issues to be resolved. Conflict between ethical and competitive behaviour may be addressed through the agreement of marketing protocols between clinicians and managers and also between purchasers and providers of health care. The aim must be to prevent fragmentation of services through the development of market shares and to ensure that the integration and collaborative philosophy of national and local health care strategies continue to take place.

Marketing and equity

A major objective of the NHS is to provide equity of health services. Frequent documentation from 1980 (Health Education Authority 1987) shows that there remain inequalities in health care locally, nationally and internationally. It is important that marketing techniques such as market research, market segmentation and marketing mix are used to identify the areas of greatest health need and to ensure that these needs are met. Whilst this is the primary role of purchasers, provider organizations also have a responsibility to their consumers to use marketing techniques in an ethical manner. It is anticipated that competition will yield efficiency gains and improve consumer choice. However, without proper controls these may well be achieved at the expense of a loss of equity and efficacy.

CONCLUSION

To accept marketing concepts into the NHS, like commercial organizations, the National Health Service will be required to make changes in management and professional attitudes, organization structure and management and professional practices. Marketing and quality management are interrelated and interdependent on one another in a consumer-driven organization. Consumer responsiveness although readily accepted by commercial organizations as an integral part of marketing, is a new and developing culture in the NHS. For the principles and techniques of marketing to be usefully applied to health care, professionals and managers will need to work together to review critically at a local level those approaches that will provide benefit both to the service and the patient.

ACTION GUIDELINES

The following guidelines are to encourage you to apply the techniques discussed in the chapter to your own clinical service:

1   Audit the service using a SWOT analysis

2   Identify which marketing techniques will be useful and develop ways of applying these to your clinical service

3 Develop a plan for marketing the service:

- ☐ promote strengths
- ☐ minimize weaknesses
- ☐ develop opportunities
- ☐ predict threats and turn them into opportunities

REFERENCES

Cavusgil S T (1986) Marketing's promise for hospitals *Business Horizons* September to October: 71.

DoH (1991) *On the State of the Public Health 1990.* London: HMSO.

Enthoven A (1985) *Reflections on the management of the National Health Service.* Occasional papers 5. London: Nuffield Provincial Hospitals Trust.

Griffiths E R (1983) Letter to the Rt Hon Norman Fowler, MP, *NHS Management Inquiry* October.

Health Education Authority (1987) *The Health Divide: Inequalities in Health in the 1980s.* London: HMSO.

Healthcare Financial Management Association (1991) *Introductory Guide to NHS Finance.* London: Healthcare Financial Management Association.

McCarthy E J (1978) *Basic Marketing: A Managerial Approach* (6th Edn). Homewood IL: Richard D Irwin Inc.

Sheaff R (1991) *Marketing for Health Services.* London: Open University Press.

FURTHER READING

Kotler P and Clarke R (1987) *Marketing for Health Care Organisations.* London: Prentice Hall.

☐ McCarthy E J (1978) *Basic Marketing: A Managerial Approach.* Homewood IL: Richard D Irwin Inc.

☐ Sheaff R (1991) *Marketing for Health Services.* London: Open University Press.

GLOSSARY

Consumer   A person or organization using the product or service, for example a patient/client or a provider unit sub-contracting services to another organization as in the case of ambulance services or tertiary services

Customer   A person or organization buying the product or service from a provider organization, for example a health care purchaser, that is a GP fundholder or DHA

Inputs   Inputs are the human and material resources committed to or used by the organization to undertake work.

Milestones   Identifiable and controllable pieces of work to be reached in a given timespan. These are particularly useful to monitor the progress of implementation

Network   Communication channels. 'Networking' is a term used to describe the sharing of information and good practice throughout the service

Organization development   A planned approach to improving the effectiveness of the whole organization

Output   The end product, e.g. an operation, a test, treatment

Process   A series of activities which taken together enable work to be carried out

Product   An object produced for consumption, usually related to manufacturing

Productivity   Effectiveness of work effort

Provider   An organization that provides a service, e.g., community units, hospitals, GPs, and non NHS organizations that provide health-related services

Purchaser   An organization that buys a service (e.g., DHA, GP Fundholder)

Reprofile   To profile a service means to outline or describe its characteristics; to reprofile will be to make recommendations for restructuring if the original profile no longer meets service requirements

Risk management   The systematic management of potential or identified risks to an organization's work to ensure that the risks are minimized or eradicated

Service   The provision of intangible (respect, dignity) and tangible (treatments) activities which provide benefit for people in need of health care

Stakeholder   Individual or group that has a personal or professional interest in the outcome

Strategy   Defines the planned growth and direction of an organization or function of an organization

Strategic management   Management of activities at a global level to ensure the strategy is achieved

Operational management   Management of activities on a day-to-day basis.

INDEX